The Scholarship of Practice: Academic-Practice Collaborations for Promoting Occupational Therapy

The Scholarship of Practice: Academic-Practice Collaborations for Promoting Occupational Therapy has been co-published simultaneously as *Occupational Therapy in Health Care*, Volume 19, Numbers 1/2 2005.

Monographic Separates from *Occupational Therapy in Health Care*™

For additional information on these and other Haworth Press titles, including descriptions, tables of contents, reviews, and prices, use the QuickSearch catalog at http://www.HaworthPress.com.

The Scholarship of Practice: Academic-Practice Collaborations for Promoting Occupational Therapy, edited by Patricia Crist, PhD, OTR/L, FAOTA, and Gary Kielhofner, DrPH, OTR, FAOTA (Vol. 19, No. 1/2, 2005). *"An excellent resource for any program pursuing collaborative, creative, and emerging practice opportunities. . . . Provides specific methods for a wide variety of applications. A must-read text!" (Kerry Muehler, MS, OTR/L, Assistant Professor and Academic Fieldwork Coordinator, Department of Occupational Therapy, University of South Dakota).*

Best Practices in Occupational Therapy Education, edited by Patricia A. Crist, PhD, OTR/L, FAOTA, and Marjorie E. Scaffa, PhD, OTR, FAOTA (Vol. 18, No. 1/2, 2004). *"A valuable resource for educators. . . Provides practical examples of student learning experiences such as problem-based learning, the use of portfolios, brain teasers and online programs." (Kathleen Matuska, MPH, OTR/L, Associate Professor of Occupational Science and Occupational Therapy, College of St. Catherine, St. Paul, Minnesota)*

Occupational Therapy Practice and Research with Persons with Multiple Sclerosis, edited by Marcia Finlayson, PhD, OT(C), OTR/L (Vol. 17, No. 3/4, 2003). *Explores the complex OT issues arising from multiple sclerosis and suggests ways to enhance OT practice or research with people with MS.*

Interprofessional Collaboration in Occupational Therapy, edited by Stanley Paul, PhD, and Cindee Q. Peterson, PhD, OTR (Vol. 15, No. 3/4, 2001). *"A good source of information. . . . Introduces the reader to the concept of interprofessional collaboration, its benefits, barriers, and strategies for developing such collaboration. . . . Presents a series of research studies that show the value of interprofessional collaboration to achieve outcomes at different levels and within different service delivery models." (Dyhalma Irizarry, PhD, OTR/L, FAOTA, Director, Occupational Therapy Program, University of Puerto Rico)*

Education for Occupational Therapy in Health Care: Strategies for the New Millennium, edited by Patricia Crist, PhD, OTR/L, FAOTA, and Marjorie Scaffa, PhD, OTR/L, FAOTA (Vol. 15, No. 1/2, 2001). *"Provides truly imaginative ideas for preparing the practitioners of the near future–and not a moment too soon! It is easy to see that these authors have been outstanding clinicians. . . . they put their OT skills to work in creating these unique learning-by-doing educational packages. Especially exciting are the clever ways in which alternative sites and programs are used to provide fieldwork experiences." (Nedra P. Gillette, MEd, OTR, ScD (Hon), Director, Institute for the Study of Occupation and Health, American Occupational Therapy Foundation)*

Community Occupational Therapy Education and Practice, edited by Beth P. Velde, PhD, OTR/L, and Peggy Prince Wittman, EdD, OTR/L, FAOTA (Vol. 13, No. 3/4, 2001). *"Introduces the concept of community-based practice in non-traditional settings. Whether one is concerned with wellness and the aging process or with debilitating situations, injuries, or diseases such as homelessness, AIDS, or multiple sclerosis, this collection details the process of moving forward." (Scott D. McPhee, DrPH, OT, FAOTA, Associate Dean and Chair, School of Occupational Therapy, Belmont University, Nashville, Tennessee)*

The Scholarship of Practice: Academic-Practice Collaborations for Promoting Occupational Therapy

Patricia Crist, PhD, OTR/L, FAOTA
Gary Kielhofner, DrPH, OTR, FAOTA
Editors

The Scholarship of Practice: Academic-Practice Collaborations for Promoting Occupational Therapy has been co-published simultaneously as *Occupational Therapy in Health Care*, Volume 19, Numbers 1/2 2005.

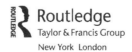

Routledge
Taylor & Francis Group
New York London

First published 2005 by The Haworth Press, Inc
10 Alice Street, Binghamton, NY 13904-1580

This edition published in 2012 by Routledge
2 Park Square, Milton Park, Abingdon, Oxon OX14 4RN
711 Third Avenue, New York, NY 10017, USA

Routledge is an imprint of the Taylor & Francis Group, an informa business

The Scholarship of Practice: Academic-Practice Collaborations for Promoting Occupational Therapy has been co-published simultaneously as *Occupational Therapy in Health Care*™, Volume 19, Numbers 1/2 2005.

The development, preparation, and publication of this work has been undertaken with great care. However, the publisher, employees, editors, and agents of The Haworth Press and all imprints of The Haworth Press, Inc., including The Haworth Medical Press® and Pharmaceutical Products Press®, are not responsible for any errors contained herein or for consequences that may ensue from use of materials or information contained in this work. Opinions expressed by the author(s) are not necessarily those of The Haworth Press, Inc. With regard to case studies, identities and circumstances of individuals discussed herein have been changed to protect confidentiality. Any resemblance to actual persons, living or dead, is entirely coincidental.

Cover design by Lora Wiggins

Library of Congress Cataloging-in-Publication Data

The scholarship of practice : academic-practice collaborations for promoting occupational therapy / Patricia Crist, Gary Kielhofner, editors.
    p. ; cm.
    Co-published simultaneously as Occupational therapy in health care, volume 19, numbers 1/2 2005.
    Includes bibliographical references and index.
    ISBN-10:   0-7890-2683-X (hard cover : alk.paper)
    ISBN-13:   978-0-7890-2683-5 (hard cover : alk.paper)
    ISBN-10:   0-7890-2684-8 (soft cover : alk.paper)
    ISBN-13:   978-0-7890-2684-2 (soft cover : alk.paper)
    1. Occupational therapy–Study and teaching. 2. Occupational therapy–Practice.
[DNLM: 1. Occupational Therapy–methods. 2. Occupational Therapy–organization & administration. 3. Interdisciplinary Communication. WB 555 S368 2005] I. Crist, Patricia A. Hickerson. II. Kielhofner, Gary, 1949-

RM735.42.S36 2005
615.8'515–dc22
                                                        2005013627

The Scholarship of Practice: Academic-Practice Collaborations for Promoting Occupational Therapy

CONTENTS

Editors' Overview   1

A Scholarship of Practice: Creating Discourse Between
Theory, Research and Practice   7
Gary Kielhofner, DrPH, OTR/L, FAOTA

ACADEMIC-PRACTICE PARTNERSHIP MODELS
AND OUTCOMES

Scholarship of Practice in the United Kingdom:
An Occupational Therapy Service Case Study   17
Kirsty Forsyth, PhD, OTR
Edward A. S. Duncan, PhD, BSc (Hons), Dip.CBT
Lynn Summerfield Mann, MSc, DipCOT

Completing the Cycle of Scholarship of Practice:
A Model for Dissemination and Utilization
of Evidence-Based Interventions   31
Elizabeth Walker Peterson, MPH, OTR/L
Elaine McMahon, MS, RN
Marianne Farkas, ScD
Jonathan Howland, PhD

A Model of University-Community Partnerships
  for Occupational Therapy Scholarship and Practice   47
    Yolanda Suarez-Balcazar, PhD
    Joy Hammel, PhD, OTR/L, FAOTA
    Christine Helfrich, PhD, OTR/L
    Jennifer Thomas
    Tom Wilson
    Daphyne Head-Ball

The Practice-Scholar Program: An Academic-Practice Partnership
  to Promote the Scholarship of "Best Practices"   71
    Patricia Crist, PhD, OTR/L, FAOTA
    Jaime Phillip Muñoz, PhD, OTR/L, FAOTA
    Anne Marie Witchger Hansen, MS, OTR/L
    Jeryl Benson, MS, OTR/L, BCP
    Ingrid Provident, EdD, OTR/L

ACADEMIC APPROACHES TO THE SCHOLARSHIP
  OF PRACTICE

Academic-Clinician Partnerships:
  A Model for Outcomes Research   95
    Karen A. Stern, EdD, OT

Synthesizing Research, Education, and Practice
  According to the Scholarship of Practice Model:
  Two Faculty Examples   107
    Renee R. Taylor, PhD
    Gail Fisher, MPA, OTR/L
    Gary Kielhofner, DrPH, OTR/L, FAOTA

A Collaborative Scholarly Project:
  Constraint-Induced Movement Therapy   123
    Jan Stube, PhD, OTR/L, BCN

New Doors: A Community Program Development Model   135
    Kathleen Swenson Miller, PhD, OTR/L
    Caryn Johnson, MS, OTR/L, FAOTA

PARTICIPATORY ACTION AND OTHER RESEARCH
METHODS APPLIED TO PRACTICE

A Participatory Action Research Approach for Identifying
Health Service Needs of Hispanic Immigrants:
Implications for Occupational Therapy   145
 Yolanda Suarez-Balcazar, PhD
 Louise I. Martinez, MPH
 Clemencia Casas-Byots, BA

Brief or New: Interagency Collaboration to Support Adults
with Developmental Disabilities in College Campus Living   165
 John F. Rose, MA, EdL
 Donna M. Heine, MA, OTR, LPC
 Cristine M. Gray, OTR

Therapists' and Clients' Perceptions of the Occupational
Performance History Interview   173
 Ashwini Apte, MS (OT), OTR
 Gary Kielhofner, DrPH, OTR/L, FAOTA
 Amy Paul-Ward, PhD
 Brent Braveman, PhD, OTR/L, FAOTA

Education and Practice Collaborations: A Pilot Case Study
Between a University Faculty and County Jail Practitioners   193
 Patricia Crist, PhD, OTR/L, FAOTA
 Andrea Fairman, MOT, OTR/L
 Jaime Phillip Muñoz, PhD, OTR/L, FAOTA
 Anne Marie Witchger Hansen, MS, OTR/L
 John Sciulli, MOT, OTR/L
 Mila Eggers, MOT, OTR/L

DEVELOPMENT OF EVIDENCE-BASED
PRACTICE SKILLS IN PRACTITIONERS

Achieving Evidence-Based Practice: A Process of Continuing
Education Through Practitioner-Academic Partnership   211
 Kirsty Forsyth, PhD, OTR
 Jane Melton, MSc, DipCOT
 Lynn Summerfield Mann, MSc, DipCOT

Index   229

ABOUT THE EDITORS

Patricia Crist, PhD, OTR/L, FAOTA, is Founding Chairperson and Professor for the Department of Occupational Therapy at Duquesne University in Pittsburgh, Pennsylvania. Dr. Crist has numerous publications including *Innovations in OT Education* (co-editor), the self-study, *Meeting the Fieldwork Challenge* (co-author), *Evaluation: Obtaining and Interpreting Data (2nd Edition)* (co-editor), and the popular *Fieldwork Issue* column in *OT Advance*. She recently co-edited *Education for Occupational Therapy in Health Care: Strategies for the New Millennium* through The Haworth Press. Dr. Crist has completed numerous scholarly works regarding fieldwork education, mental health interventions, parents with disabilities and research. Currently, she is Chairperson of the Board of Directors of the National Board for Certification in Occupational Therapy. She is a Fellow of the American Occupational Therapy Association.

Gary Kielhofner, DrPH, OTR, FAOTA, is currently Professor and Wade/Meyer Chair in the Department of Occupational Therapy at the University of Illinois at Chicago. His research focuses on a wide range of populations, but one focus is programming for persons with AIDS, mental health and substance abuse problems. Dr. Kielhofner maintains a close involvement in clinical practice, research, and consultation. He is the co-author/editor of 15 books and has published over 100 articles. Dr. Kielhofner is a Fellow of the American Occupational Therapy Association, a member of the Academy of Research of the American Occupational Therapy Foundation, and a recipient of the A. Jean Ayres award. He is also the recipient of 3 honorary Doctoral Degrees.

Editors' Overview

Innovations in health care or education are successful because an individual addresses an unmet need by envisioning new possibilities. This type of innovation requires leadership and risk-taking, coupled with a passion to do better and a hunger for a new journey.

Currently, occupational therapists are uniquely positioned to engage emerging opportunities in practice and education. However, as time passes, initial intentions are transformed into even better plans or programs as new lessons are learned and contexts are better understood. A story demonstrating the value of occupational therapy likely unfolds. In sharing the story later, still more insights and reflections emerge. Finally, the listeners or readers can be motivated from the experience of others to consider the opportunity before them.

As co-editors, our journeys into the scholarship of practice were motivated by our own reasons and we developed our approaches within the context of our own education and practice environments. Quite by accident, we came together at the 2002 World Federation of Occupational Therapy conference in Sweden. Gary presented the keynote that challenged occupational therapist scholars to partner with practitioners to develop and study practice as his faculty members do under their banner of a Scholarship of Practice at the University of Illinois-Chicago (UIC). On that same day, Pat co-presented a poster with her faculty, Anne Marie Witchger Hansen, regarding their Practice-Scholar Program at Duquesne University (DU) developing 'best practices' practitioner models which seamlessly integrated activities of scholarship in emerging innovative occupation-based practice areas along with facilitating student professional development.

[Haworth co-indexing entry note]: "Editors' Overview." Crist, Patricia, and Gary Kielhofner. Co-published simultaneously in *Occupational Therapy in Health Care* (The Haworth Press, Inc.) Vol. 19, No. 1/2, 2005, pp. 1-5; and: *The Scholarship of Practice: Academic-Practice Collaborations for Promoting Occupational Therapy* (ed: Patricia Crist, and Gary Kielhofner) The Haworth Press, Inc., 2005, pp. 1-5. Single or multiple copies of this article are available for a fee from The Haworth Document Delivery Service [1-800-HAWORTH, 9:00 a.m. - 5:00 p.m. (EST). E-mail address: docdelivery@haworthpress.com].

doi:10.1300/J003v19n01_01

A brief conversation at the airport between us waiting for our return trip to the USA indicated that while our approaches were different, we shared a common interest to lead new approaches to the study of occupational therapy practice through partnerships and demonstrate possible practitioner roles and activities to embed the study of practice as part of everyday work.

The Fall 2003 program director's workshop highlighting the UIC approach to the scholarship of practice, resulted in immense interest from many program directors to pursue the concept of the scholarship of practice. Each inquiry was curious about how to adapt the scholarship of practice to support their own missions, academic contexts and faculty abilities to pursue scholarship through practice partnerships. Several were intrigued by the opportunities emerging from a different approach that Duquesne University was taking because of the nature of their academic and community content and resources. A formal meeting between the UIC and DU faculties at this Program Director's meeting in Chicago in Fall 2003 resulted in Anne Dickerson, Editor of *OTHC*, approving our proposal to move forward with a special publication on the scholarship of practice. Clearly from our various activities, educators and practitioners were ready to embrace the scholarship of practice and were curious to learn from the experiences of others who are pioneering this approach. Thus, our primary objective is to highlight current approaches that close the gap between scholarship and practice.

In occupational therapy, when investigators and practitioners work together to combine innovation with action, documentation and reflection, they embark on a journey that is the scholarship of practice. The scholarship of practice in occupational therapy will take on many different forms that reflect the unique needs of the academic and practice settings; no 'one size fits all' because the scholarship of practice in occupational therapy is built on unique partnerships between the academic and practice settings. Each brings their own mission and purpose for seeking the partnership and the partnership develops and sustains itself only when mutual interest and needs are addressed.

As we compared notes on the evolution of our two different scholarship of practice approaches, we become aware that faculty in an occupational therapy education program in a research intensive program will have different motivations for engaging in the scholarship of practice than one will in a teaching intensive setting. Likewise, practice partners vary in their contexts and missions for practice. Thus, multiple Scholarship of Practice models can emerge, each providing a model for others to understand and even replicate. We proceeded with an open call for papers for this volume, realizing that few scholarship of practice models probably existed at this point in time. The authors felt that it was important to provide readers with the greatest variety of approaches possible. This variety would stimulate even more models to emerge in the future.

OVERVIEW

The primary goals of this special publication were to:

- discuss the reasons for the gaps between scholarship and practice
- highlight how scholarship can support the validity of occupational therapy practice through investigations studying everyday practice grounded in the reality of therapeutic encounters
- demonstrate how the engagement of occupations allows our clients, patients, etc., to reclaim their lives in the face of illness or disability
- illustrate models of practice-based research that can be implemented to provide evidence regarding the efficacy of occupational therapy services and approaches

The editors wish to thank the authors who submitted manuscripts to achieve this goal. Inside this volume, you will find rich pragmatic descriptions of academic-practice partnership models and outcome in four different contexts. This section is followed by faculty from four different universities or colleges outlining academic approaches to facilitate the scholarship of practice. The third section focuses on four examples of research methods that have been applied successfully in practice settings to develop evidence to support the practice of occupational therapy. In the last section, a group of authors provide a model to develop evidence-based practice competencies among practitioners to apply daily during intervention planning and overall program development.

We hope that the papers presented in this publication stimulate a growing interest by more occupational therapy and faculty practitioners to focus on the scholarship of practice. Evidence to describe the specific contribution of occupational therapy as a profession is critical to retaining our value as an essential service in our practice settings. Further, we need models to follow in practice that embed scholarship as part of everyday practice. Creating meaningful databases from individual responses to occupational therapy interventions can ultimately lead to studies demonstrating the validity of occupational therapy intervention. Accumulation of these practice studies will validate to others the importance of occupational therapy services. In closing, one of the greatest challenges that occupational therapy faces today is creating a new approach to patient documentation that lends itself to demonstrate the specific impact of occupation-based interventions. Global program evaluation may demonstrate benefits of a program through measures such as length of stay, recidivism, and overall functional change. However, this approach frequently leaves occupational therapy practitioners to demonstrate the specific outcomes from occupational therapy. We encourage faculty-practitioner teams to come together and delineate systematic, reasonable approaches to patient or client assessment and re-assessment. This simple habit would create a wealth of scholarship regarding the efficacy and effectiveness of occupational therapy practice ensuring our future and most importantly, our patients' enhanced quality of life resulting from the application of evidence to everyday practice.

IT TAKES A COMMUNITY TO ...

The review of journal articles was provided by a cadre of invited individuals from both practice and education from across the United States as well as Scotland and England. I want to thank them for their beneficial services, as their analysis and feed- back underpinned the selection process. Thanks to each of you for volunteering.

Anita Atwal	Patti LaVesser
Erna Imperatore Blanche	Anne MacRae
Alfred G. Bracciano	Jane Melton
Brent Braveman	Jaime Muñoz
Sara Brayman	Peggy Neufeld
Catana Brown	Frances Oakley
Regina Michael Campbell	Ingrid Provident
Christine Craik	Charlotte Royeen
Cathy Dolhi	Marian K. Scheinholtz
Linda Florey	Sally Schultz
Kirsty Forsyth	Karen C. Spencer
Daniel Goldreich	Ronald G. Stone
Joy Hammel	Yolanda Suarez-Balcazar
DeLana Honaker	Deborah Walens

Thanks to each of you for giving of yourself as reviewers this past year.

IN CLOSING

As the editors of this special edition regarding the scholarship of practice, we urge faculty and practitioners to create their own scholarship of practice through being a practice-scholar. We firmly believe that the Scholarship of Practice will be the norm, not the exception.

Patricia Crist, PhD, OTR/L, FAOTA
Gary Kielhofner, DrPH, OTR, FAOTA
Volume Editors

A Scholarship of Practice:
Creating Discourse Between
Theory, Research and Practice

Gary Kielhofner, DrPH, OTR/L, FAOTA

SUMMARY. Occupational therapy has experienced a tremendous growth both of theory and research. However, there is little evidence that this renaissance of knowledge has been paralleled by changes in practice. Instead, academics tend to express concern that practice lags behind scholarship while clinicians bemoan the irrelevance of theory and research to their everyday work. This paper discusses the scholarship of practice. This approach is based on the assumption that those who ultimately will use the knowledge must be partners in its generation. Thus, it emphasizes cooperative efforts in which practitioners and scholars work together as partners to advance both knowledge and practice. *[Article copies available for a fee from The Haworth Document Delivery Service: 1-800-HAWORTH. E-mail address: <docdelivery@haworthpress.com> Website: <http://www.HaworthPress.com> © 2005 by The Haworth Press, Inc. All rights reserved.]*

KEYWORDS. Theory, scholarship of practice, knowledge generation, participatory action research, knowledge-creating systems, empowerment evaluation

Gary Kielhofner is affiliated with the University of Illinois at Chicago, Department of Occupational Therapy, 1919 West Taylor Street, Chicago, IL 60612-7250.

[Haworth co-indexing entry note]: "A Scholarship of Practice: Creating Discourse Between Theory, Research and Practice." Kielhofner, Gary. Co-published simultaneously in *Occupational Therapy in Health Care* (The Haworth Press, Inc.) Vol. 19, No. 1/2, 2005, pp. 7-16; and: *The Scholarship of Practice: Academic-Practice Collaborations for Promoting Occupational Therapy* (ed: Patricia Crist, and Gary Kielhofner) The Haworth Press, Inc., 2005, pp. 7-16. Single or multiple copies of this article are available for a fee from The Haworth Document Delivery Service [1-800-HAWORTH, 9:00 a.m. - 5:00 p.m. (EST). E-mail address: docdelivery@haworthpress.com].

Available online at http://www.haworthpress.com/web/OTHC
doi:10.1300/J003v19n01_02

THE SCHOLARSHIP PRACTICE GAP

In the last quarter century, occupational therapy has experienced something of an explosion of scholarship. Tremendous growth both of theory and research in the field has resulted in a wealth of new concepts and evidence in the field. Much of the theoretical work and research has sought to better envision the role of occupation in health and well-being and its role as a therapeutic tool.

Unfortunately, there is little evidence that this renaissance of knowledge has been paralleled by a renaissance of practice. Instead academics tend to express concern that practice lags behind scholarship while clinicians bemoan the irrelevance of theory and research to their everyday work.

Why might practitioners not find theory and research relevant to their everyday work? It is likely that many factors account for this, including the demands and constraints of practice settings that leave limited time for reflection and innovation. However, an overlooked factor is how the occupational therapy generates knowledge and the resulting form that the field's knowledge takes.

Most of the new knowledge that gets produced and disseminated (i.e., published, presented at conferences) are the result of academics or graduate students working under academics. The kinds of concerns that these persons address when they are developing concepts or conducting investigations revolve around logical and rigor. What they too often ignore or consider secondary is relevance. That is, the question of what constitutes good knowledge for practice takes a back seat to academic concerns for conceptual and methodological rigor.

Recognizing this as a universal problem in the professions, writers such as Barnett (1994), Eraut (1994), and MacKinnon (1991) argue that, rather than de-coupling knowledge generation and knowledge use, these activities should be tied together into a single enterprise. Achieving this aim is not simple however, since a number of barriers exist. One barrier to coupling scholarship and practice is the fact that those who are generating knowledge and those who use knowledge work in different types of institutions (universities and colleges versus hospitals, rehabilitation centers, nursing homes and school systems with different agendas and expectations). A second barrier is the "everyday worlds" in which these two constituents operate. Academics work in a world where knowledge is judged, as noted above, by scientific rigor and where the ultimate legitimization of knowledge is publication. Practitioners exist in a world where knowledge is judged by what it allows them to do and the practical results it generates. Such institutional and pragmatic barriers, mean that coupling scholarship and practice into a meaningful relationship requires innovative new models.

A Scholarship of Practice

One successful model of profitably coupling scholarship and practice is the concept of a scholarship of practice (Hammel, Finlayson, Kielhofner, Helfrich, & Peterson, 2002; Kielhofner, 2001, 2004) which first emerged at the University of Illinois at Chicago (UIC). A key element of the scholarship of practice is that in a profession such as occupational therapy legitimate scholarship is devoted to improve practice. While scholarship that aims to improve practice, routinely generates new knowledge, it does not seek to generate knowledge for its own sake. Rather, knowledge is valued because it enhances practice and practice outcomes. This is an important distinction since scholarship in academic circles traditionally emphasized the importance of knowledge for its own sake. Claims that such knowledge might inform or benefit practice are not seen as sufficient for legitimizing inquiry that does not directly address questions of concern or interest to practice.

The scholarship of practice was originally defined as "a dialectic in which theoretical and empirical knowledge is brought to bear on the practical problems of therapeutic work and in which the latter raise questions to be addressed through scholarship." The aim of the scholarship of practice was stated to better understand the needs of people that occupational therapy serves, and the ways in which we can most effectively address these needs (Kielhofner, 2001). As such it includes research that:

- Identifies problems and needs that can be addressed by OT
- Develops assessment measures of targeted client outcomes
- Illuminates therapeutic processes
- Tests therapeutic strategies or programs
- Investigates OT contributions to interdisciplinary programs (Kielhofner, 2001)

Hammel, Finlayson, Kielhofner, Helfrich, and Peterson (2001) identified the following key elements of a scholarship of practice:

- Commitment to conducting research that directly responds to and contributes to practice

- Partnerships with individuals and organizations outside of the academic department to create new educational, practice and research opportunities,
- Creating synergies to advance practice and scholarship simultaneously

This approach is based on the assumption that those who ultimately will use the knowledge must be partners in its generation. The scholarship of practice, thus, begins with the premise that researchers and theorists in the field must work together with practitioners to not only generate the field's theory and research but also to advance practice. Consequently, the scholarship of practice emphasizes that:

- occupational therapy knowledge should grow out of collaboration between those in academic and practice roles.
- the collaboration must be a true partnership in which power is shared between academics and practitioners so that the perspectives that characterize the "everyday worlds" of each are fully represented.

In such a collaborative model, scholarship provides tools to enhance understanding of practice problems (e.g., methodological principles and rules for verifying knowledge). Practice points to what we should know and, by applying theory to real life, enriches the understanding and development of theory. In such a collaborative model, the theoretical, empirical and practical are interwoven. Knowledge becomes not simply knowledge about something, but knowledge of how to do something. It is a new form of knowledge-in-action. This, in short, is the guiding vision of a scholarship of practice. The next critical component is creating specific ways of operationalizing this vision.

Interdisciplinary Models of Cooperative Knowledge Generation

The scholarship of practice has also been informed by interdisciplinary models of developing knowledge relevant to solving real-world problems. Variously called participatory action research, empowerment evaluation, and knowledge-generating systems, these approaches all articulate principles and strategies for the involvement those who engage in or receive professional services in research that is designed to generate information for practice.

Participatory action research. Participatory action research has its origins in third-world social activism (Townsend, Birch, Langley, & Langille, 2000; Friere, 1993). It combines investigation and action to define and address local problems (Brown & Tandon, 1983).

When used in the context of developing and evaluating services, PAR aims to assure that the services and how they are evaluated reflect the perspectives of providers and consumers. PAR seeks to accomplish this aim by involving such stakeholders as true partners who have an active role in shaping services and identifying the criteria or standards against which effective service should be judged (Balcazar, Keys, Kaplan, & Suarez-Balcazar, 1998, Taylor, Hammel, & Braveman, 2004).

PAR is not a research method per se, but rather an approach that maximizes the involvement of stakeholders. It is typically associated with action-oriented projects that emphasize the achievement of local, consumer-driven goals over the traditional aims of positivist science (Bradbury & Reason, 2001; Boyce & Lysack, 2000). Therefore, much of the literature highlights differences between PAR approaches and more traditional research that only emphasizes prevailing standards of scientific rigor. This research approach has been noted to produce findings of greater relevance and social validity. Notably, because stakeholders are involved in shaping it, they are more likely to use and to benefit from the knowledge generated in the research (Brown, 1991; Tewey, 1997; Krogh, 1998).

Taylor, Hammel, and Braveman (2004) discuss and provide examples of how PAR can be used within studies that aim to develop and test occupational therapy service. They note that while approaches to studying services are limited to professionally-generated, intellectual ways of knowing, PAR embraces different kinds of knowing that can provide important evidence about practice. They also emphasize the importance of involving therapists and consumers in the research process.

Empowerment Evaluation

Empowerment evaluation (EE) builds upon and shares principles with PAR. However, it focuses on enabling local groups or communities to create and/or evaluate programs. EE encapsulates the philosophy that knowledge to inform practice should be generated in an interactive context where investigation, practice, and innovation are linked together (Fawcett, Paine-Andrews, Francisco, Scultz, Richter, Lewis, Williams, Harris, Berkley, Fisher, & Lopez, 1995; Fetterman, 1996; Suarez-Balcazar & Harper, 2003).

Empowerment evaluation ordinarily links knowing and doing through a cyclical process of investigation, education, and action. As information is gathered, it is analyzed and applied to enhance services and the results of changed service are then evaluated and the cycle continues. Empowerment Evaluation models (Suarez-Balcazar & Harper, 2003; Fawcett, Boothroyd, Schultz, Francisco, Carson & Bremby, 2003) stress that:

- EE is an emergent process that cannot be determined and structured beforehand like traditional research designs that emphasize control by the researcher.
- The academic is present in the evaluation not as an expert to pass judgment but as a facilitator to enable community partners to take control of the development and evaluation of their own programs.
- Academics and the community members with whom they form a partnership may take turns filling roles such as coach, educator, or technical assistant.
- EE is a capacity building process in which local stakeholders engage in learning by doing.

Benefits of EE are that staff and others in the agencies whose programs are evaluated are more likely to respond to and use the information generated through evaluation and that the local personnel involved in the evaluation learn new skills for creating, evaluating, and securing resources for their services (Suarez-Balcazar, Orellana-Damacela, Portillo, Sharma, & Lanum, 2004).

Knowledge Creating Systems

PAR and Empowerment Evaluation stress inquiry in which the primary aim of research is to generate locally-desired and utilizable knowledge and building capacity of local stakeholders. Senge and Scharmer (2001), building on PAR and EE concepts, propose an approach that incorporate both the focus on addressing local problem and building capacity while at the same time creating generalizable knowledge of the kind emphasized in traditional research. In their approach all three of these aims are incorporated into "a knowledge-creating system." This system is a community of researchers and practitioners who work together to create theory, along with practical tools and know-how.

Consequently a knowledge creating system involves three interacting domains of activity:

- capacity-building,
- practice innovation, and
- research.

Capacity-building aims to enhance local stakeholders' awareness and capabilities both as individuals and collectively. This element of the knowledge-creating system results in practical knowledge among the participants. Practice innovation involves creating a new vision of what can be accomplished in practice and going on to create the practical tools and approaches that achieve the vision. Practice innovation aims often create tools that not only work in the situation at hand, but that can also be used in other comparable situations. According to Senge and Scharmer (p. 240), research is a "disciplined approach to discovery and understanding, with a commitment to share what is learned." Thus, research aims to create generalizable, theoretical knowledge.

The knowledge creating system aims to integrate all three types of knowledge creation and use within a single community of people working together. Thus concepts, evidence, and practice innovations are created at the same time that practitioners' knowledge of and use of these resources is increased. All participants share a commitment to all three goals. For example, practitioners are involved in the process of creating generalizable knowledge, while academics are involved in solving practice problems. In this knowledge-creating system the traditional equal weight is given to generating knowledge and applying it, since these activities are inseparable. Kielhofner (2005) and Forsyth, Summerfield-Mann, and Kielhofner (2005) have described how such knowledge creating systems can be created in occupational therapy through academic practitioner collaboration.

While the ideas of PAR, EE, and KCS are each unique, taken together they indicate that knowledge development best occurs when:

- Those who ultimately will use the knowledge should be involved in helping to generate and refine it
- Knowledge generation should be grounded in the kinds of contexts in which it is designed for application
- Knowledge generation should emerge from cooperation and teamwork between those whose primary roles are to generate knowledge and those whose roles involve application of knowledge
- The desire to generate generalizable knowledge (theoretical and empirical) is balanced with the desire to create local problem-solutions and technical know-how

REFERENCES

Balcazar, F. E., Keys, C. B., & Garate-Serafini, S. (1995). Learning to recruit assistance to attain transition goals: A program for adjudicated youth with disabilities. *Remedial and Special Education, 16,* 237-246.

Balcazar, F. E., Keys, C. B., Kaplan, D. L., Suarez-Balcazar, Y. (1998). Participatory action research and people with disabilities: Principles and challenges. *Canadian Journal of Rehabilitation, 12,* 105-112.

Barnett, R. (1994) The Limits of Competence Knowledge, Higher Education and Society. Society for Research into Higher Education & Open University Press.

Barnett, R. (1997). Higher occupational education: A critical business. *The Society for Research into Higher Education.* UK: Open University Press.

Boyce, W. & Lysack, C. (2000). Community participation: Uncovering its meanings in CBR. In Thomas, M. & Thomas, M.J. (2000). *Selected readings in Community Based Rehabilitation: CBR in transition (Series 1).* Bangalore: *Asia Pacific Disability Rehabilitation Journal.*

Boyer, E. L. (1990). *Scholarship reconsidered: Priorities of the professorate.* Princeton, NJ: The Carnegie Foundation for the Advancement of Teaching. *American Journal of Occupational Therapy, 45 (4),* 300-310.

Bradbury, H., & Reason. P. (2001). Conclusion: Broadening the bandwidth of validity: Issues and choice-points for improving the quality of action research. In P. Reason & Bradbury, H. (Eds.). *Handbook of Action Research: Participative Inquiry and Practice.* London: Sage.

Brown, D. L., & Tandon, R. (1983). Ideology and political economy in inquiry: Action research and participatory research. *Journal of Applied Behavioral Science, 19,* 277-294.

Brown, E. (1991). Community action for health promotion: A strategy to empower individuals and communities. *International Journal of Health Services, 21,* 441-456.

David, J., Zakus, L., & Lysack, C. L. (1998). Revisiting community participation. *Health policy and planning, 13* (1), 1-12.

Dickoff, J., James. P., & Wiedenbach, E. (1968). Theory in a practice discipline. *Nursing Research, 17,* 415-435.

Eraut, M. (1994) Developing Professional Knowledge and Competence. Washington. Falmer Press.

Fawcett, S. B., Paine-Andrews, A., Francisco, V. T., Scultz, J. A., Richter, K. P., Lewis, R. K., Williams, E. L., Harris. K. J., Berkley. J. Y., Fisher, J. L., & Lopez, C. M. (1995). Using empowerment theory in collaborative partnerships for community mental health and development. *American Journal of Community Psychology, 23,* (5), 677-697.

Fawcett, S. B., Boothroyd, R., Schultz. J. A., Francisco, V. T., Carson, V., & Bremby, R. (2003). Building Capacity for participatory evaluation within community initiatives. In Suarez-Balcazar. Y. and Harper, G. W. (editors) *Empowerment and Participatory Evaluation of Community Interventions.* New York: The Haworth Press, Inc.

Fetterman, D. M. (1996). Empowerment evaluation: An introduction to theory and practice. In *Empowerment Evaluation: Knowledge and tools for self-assessment and accountability*. D. M. Fetterman, S. J. Kaftarian & A. Wandersman Ed. Thousand Oaks California: Sage.

Forsyth, K. Summerfield-Mann, L., & Kielhofner, G. (2005) A Scholarship of practice: Making occupation-focused, theory-driven, evidence-based practice a reality. *British Journal of Occupational Therapy*, 68, 261-268.

Freire, P. (1993). *Pedagogy of the Oppressed*. New York: Herder and Herder.

Hammel, J., Finlayson, M., Kielhofner, G., Helfrich, C., & Peterson, E. (2002). Educating scholars of practice: An approach to preparing tomorrow's researchers. *Occupational Therapy in Health Care, 15 (1/2)*, 157-176.

Heron, J. (1988). Validity in co-operative inquiry. In *Human Inquiry in Action*. P. Reason (Ed.). Sage Publications: London.

Kielhofner, G. (2001) A scholarship of practice. Paper presented at the American Occupational Therapy Foundation Colloquium and Tea at the American Occupational Therapy Association Conference.

Kielhofner, G. (2004) *Conceptual Foundations of Occupational Therapy* (3rd ed.). Philadelphia: F.A. Davis.

Kielhofner, G. (2005). Scholarship and Practice: Bridging the Divide. *American Journal of Occupational Therapy, 59*, 231-239.

Krogh, K. (1995) Developing a partnership agreement. In J. Pivik (Ed.), *Facilitating collaborative research between consumers and researchers*. (pp. 69-75). Ottawa, ON: Institute for Rehabilitation Research and Development.

Krogh, K. (1998). A conceptual framework of community partnerships: Perspective of people with disabilities on power, beliefs and values. *Canadian Journal of Rehabilitation, 12* (2), 123-134.

MacKinnon, C. (1991). From practice to theory, or what is a white women anyway? *Yale Journal of Law and Feminism, 4 (13)*, 13-22.

Mattingly, C., & Fleming, M. H. (1994). *Clinical reasoning: Forms of inquiry in a therapeutic practice*. Philadelphia, PA: F. A. Davis.

Maxwell, N. (1992). What kind of inquiry can best help us create a good world? *Science, Technology, & Human Values, 17*, 205-227.

McColl, M. A., Law, M., & Stewart, D. (1993). *Theoretical basis of occupational therapy*. Thorofare, NJ: Slack, Inc.

Minkler, M. (1985). Building supportive ties and sense of community among the inner-city elderly: The Tenderloin senior outreach project. *Health Education Quarterly, 12*, 303-314.

Reason, P. (1988). The co-operative inquiry group. In *Human Inquiry in Action*. P. Reason (Ed.) Sage Publications: London.

Suarez-Balcazar, Y. and Harper, G. W. (Eds.) (2003) *Empowerment and Participatory Evaluation of Community Interventions*. New York: The Haworth Press, Inc.

Suarez-Balcazar, Y. & Harper, G. W. (2003) Community-based approaches to empowerment and participatory evaluation. In Suarez-Balcazar, Y. and Harper, G. W. (editors) *Empowerment and Participatory Evaluation of Community Interventions*. New York: The Haworth Press, Inc.

Suarez-Balcazar, Y., Orellana-Damacela, L., Portillo, N., Sharma, A., & Lanum, M. (2003) Implementing an Outcomes model in the participatory evaluation of community initiatives. In Suarez-Balcazar, Y. and Harper, G. W. (editors) *Empowerment and*

Participatory Evaluation of Community Interventions. New York: The Haworth Press, Inc.

Taylor, R., Braveman, B., & Hammel, J. (2004) Developing and Evaluating community services through Participatory Action Research: Two case examples *American Journal of Occupational Therapy 58*, 35-43.

Tewey, B. P. (1997) Building participatory action research partnerships in disability and rehabilitation research. National Institute on Disability and Rehabilitation Research.

Townsend, E., Birch, D. E., Langley, J., & Langille, L. (2000). Participatory research in a mental health clubhouse. *Occupational Therapy Journal of Research, 20*, 18-44.

ACADEMIC-PRACTICE PARTNERSHIP
MODELS AND OUTCOMES

Scholarship of Practice
in the United Kingdom:
An Occupational Therapy
Service Case Study

Kirsty Forsyth, PhD, OTR
Edward A. S. Duncan, PhD, BSc (Hons), Dip.CBT
Lynn Summerfield Mann, MSc, DipCOT

Kirsty Forsyth is Director, UK Centre for Outcomes Research and Education (UKCORE), London South Bank University, London, and Senior Lecturer, Queen Margaret University College, Edinburgh. Edward A. S. Duncan is Postdoctoral Research Fellow, Nursing Midwifery and Allied Health Professions Research Unit, The University of Stirling, Stirling, and Clinical Specialist Occupational Therapist, The State Hospital, Carstairs, Lanarkshire. Lynn Summerfield Mann is Principal Lecturer, Occupational Therapy Post Graduate Programme and Co-Director, UK Centre for Outcomes Research and Education (UKCORE), London South Bank University, London.

The authors would like to acknowledge the stakeholders involved in the UKCORE/TSH partnership. They would also like to acknowledge Susan Prior, Orchard Clinic, Royal Edinburgh Hospital for her support with Figure 2.

[Haworth co-indexing entry note]: "Scholarship of Practice in the United Kingdom: An Occupational Therapy Service Case Study." Forsyth, Kirsty, Edward A. S. Duncan, and Lynn Summerfield Mann. Co-published simultaneously in *Occupational Therapy in Health Care* (The Haworth Press, Inc.) Vol. 19, No. 1/2, 2005, pp. 17-29; and: *The Scholarship of Practice: Academic-Practice Collaborations for Promoting Occupational Therapy* (ed: Patricia Crist, and Gary Kielhofner) The Haworth Press, Inc., 2005, pp. 17-29. Single or multiple copies of this article are available for a fee from The Haworth Document Delivery Service [1-800-HAWORTH, 9:00 a.m. - 5:00 p.m. (EST). E-mail address: docdelivery@haworthpress.com].

SUMMARY. Occupational therapy is required to deliver and generate evidence-based practice. This paper illustrates an approach to meeting these evidence-based expectations. Specifically, there is a description of the development of a partnership between the United Kingdom Centre for Outcomes Research and Education (UKCORE) and The State Hospital which is a forensic mental health service. This case study will illuminate (a) a rationale for partnership, (b) the process of building the partnership, and (c) outcomes of the partnership. Principles of scholarship of practice will be identified and ways of supporting services to integrate occupational therapy knowledge generation and utilisation will be outlined. *[Article copies available for a fee from The Haworth Document Delivery Service: 1-800-HAWORTH. E-mail address: <docdelivery@haworthpress.com> Website: <http://www.HaworthPress.com> © 2005 by The Haworth Press, Inc. All rights reserved.]*

KEYWORDS. Occupation, theory, evidence-based practice

BACKGROUND AND RATIONALE

Introduction

Occupational therapy endorses the importance of research findings in shaping practice (Humphries et al., 2000; Metcalf et al., 2001; Bennett et al., 2003). An accessible evidence-base would support practitioners in their clinical decision-making, empowering occupational therapists to review the way in which they have traditionally carried out their practice. Furthermore, it has been argued, evidence-based practice can help clinicians influence service purchasers and managers to provide occupation-focused intervention as part of health care for clients.

However, there is a growing consensus that, many clinicians feel unable to use evidence to support practice. It has been argued that occupational therapy lacks the research capacity to respond systematically and existing research in the field tends to be sporadic rather than strategically planned (HEFCE, 2001; Creek & Ilott, 2002). Creek (2003:27) suggested that experienced occupational therapists use a wide range of techniques that ". . . appear to work rather than appraising the research evidence." Metcalf et al. (2001:436) stated that only 5.8% of the occupational therapists in their study reported ". . . any interest in finding and reading research." McCluskey and Cusick (2002) reported occupational therapists were aware they needed to change their practice but didn't know how or where to start.

Identified barriers to building research capacity include workload pressures, lack of protected time, inadequate arrangements to provide cover whilst clinicians carry out research, lack of support for therapists, and the failure to develop research leaders and establish research career pathways (HEFEC, 2001; Creek & Ilott, 2002). Despite the challenges involved, research has the potential to generate recognition of the valuable contribution occupational therapy can make to improve health (Godfrey, 2000). Reasons for this apparent lack of research productivity needed to be explored and solutions identified. This paper will outline a scholarship of practice approach to supporting a mental health service tackle these challenging issues in order to embed evidence into practice while simultaneously generating evidence for practice.

The State Hospital

The State Hospital (TSH) is a high security hospital that caters for offenders with mental disorders. TSH is a national service for Scotland and Northern Ireland and receives referrals from the National Health Service, prisons and court. In 1991, TSH became the first high security hospital to employ state-registered occupational therapists. The service uses the Model of Human Occupation (MOHO) as its primary conceptual model, guiding clinicians' formulation of a client's difficulties, assessment, and intervention. Occupational therapy services are provided to improve engagement in occupation within the hospital in preparation for clients' future discharge.

The TSH occupational therapy service was experiencing some of the barriers to evidence based practice described in the broader literature. Despite a managerial commitment to delivering research outcomes, there were challenges to strategically building evidence. Research outcomes were developed in an *ad hoc* fashion and according to personal interest. Although occupational therapy managers were supportive of clinicians undertaking research, practitioners perceived it as an added extra to clinical work. As a result, little research was actually carried out within the service that had a significant impact on future service delivery (Duncan et al., 2004). Therefore, whilst there was verbal support for research in practice, the lack of a strategy to develop appropriate systems of data gathering within practice resulted in little research occurring. This appeared to frustrate staff. A review of the occupational therapy department commitment to research in practice came when the individual who had been supplying academic supervision for the staff was no longer able to continue in her role. The occupational therapy service realized that managerial support and quality academic supervision were not in themselves sufficient to enable clinicians to undertake sustainable research studies that have an effect on clinical practice. The department then approached the staff of the UK Centre for Outcomes Research and Education (UKCORE), as they were gaining a positive reputation for overcoming exactly the types of challenges that were inhibiting the department from progressing with research in practice as they desired. This paper describes the process of the collaboration between TSH and UKCORE.

UKCORE

- The UKCORE was originally built in collaboration with and built on principles from the scholarship of practice (Kielhofner, 2005) Centre for Outcomes Research and Education at the University of Illinois at Chicago (Kielhofner et al., 2004). The UKCORE was built on a scholarship of practice philosophy and was viewed as an organizational structure to bring together academic departments and occupational therapy practice settings (see Figure 1). The centre began working with several occupational therapy services in the greater London area in England. The focus of such collaborations were to develop theory driven, evidence base practice through the collaboration of academics and clinicians, working in partnership. Amongst other aims, the centre strives to help practitioners integrate evidence into their work and to incorporate the generation of further evidence as a core part of their work.

The UKCORE is now based at London South Bank University, and involves ongoing relationships with occupational therapy services in London, Gloucestershire and Lanarkshire. The UKCORE works to integrate scholarship (i.e., research and theory development), education, and practice across each organizational settings.

PROCESS OF BUILDING SCHOLARSHIP OF PRACTICE

The State Hospital in Partnership with UKCORE

As previously discussed, practitioners at TSH tended to view research as something separate from their everyday work. This was not

FIGURE 1. UK Centre for Outcomes Research and Education (UKCORE)

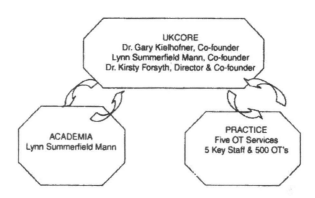

due to a reluctance to participate in research, but rather because the predominant model of research was one in which the links between the clinicians role and theory development was not explicit. The first step, therefore, was to assess how best to introduce research into practice and to consider how to contribute to research in a way that would have a positive impact on the everyday practice and experience of the clinicians. This was a daunting challenge, as it required the clinicians to view research in a radically different way than they previously had. Their first goal of the new partnership between TSH and UKCORE was therefore to change the research-practice culture within the service. This required the service to reconsider how it perceived and used MOHO in practice; a re-evaluation of the focus of the services interventions to ensure that they were evidence-based and occupation-focused; and to commence the redevelopment of the service so that it enabled clinicians to gather data for research studies as a routine part of the clinicians' practice. All of this has required a great deal of attention to be paid to supporting clinicians to change from established clinical routines to a more evidence-based culture.

(i) Initial Negotiations

The partnership between The State Hospital and UKCORE began with examining the possibility of generating new roles and structures. The work required a new system of relationships with people taking non-traditional roles and activities. Specifically, this means that academics (educators, researchers, and students) and practice (clinicians, clients, and administrators) all take on roles within this new system and with an appreciation of the different constituencies and how they relate to each other.

The goal was to have both academics and practitioners working together as "practice scholars" who are jointly involved in the development of the evidence-base for occupational therapy. Importantly, each staff group has had to learn how to do things differently. For the clinicians, there were new evidence-based assessments to consider and implement, as well as getting used to working in collaboration with academics and viewing the developments within the service as the focus of this new partnership. For the academics, it was important to understand how the clinicians worked within a secure environment. This was an important initial stage of outlining the working relationship that set the context within which the work was to be completed.

(ii) Building Structures to Support Delivering of Evidence-Based Practice

It is necessary to understand the perspectives of all stakeholders in the system before attempting to implement changes in practice (Grol, 1997). It is important to develop routine mechanisms by which individual and organisational change can occur (NHS Centre for Reviews and Dissemination, 1999; FoNS, 2001). Indeed, building research infrastructures and capacity are commonly identified as areas for urgent attention in the UK (Scottish Executive, 2002). UKCORE has, therefore, supported TSH to develop several structures to support the change process. These structures evolved from ongoing dialogues between stakeholders about what was required to deliver occupation focused, theory driven, evidence-based practice at TSH. They included (a) strategic planning, (b) managerial structures, and (c) evidence-based development groups for staff. These are briefly described below.

(a) Strategic Planning. Strategic planning is important to support any change process (Fitzgerald et al., 2003). This was specifically identified by TSH as a high priority. TSH staff felt their previous attempts at research had not been strategically planned and therefore was not cumulatively building research over time. Strategic plans could very clearly identify the priorities for TSH services and how resources should be focused. UKCORE and TSH worked together to identify and develop the parameters of the service and an R&D strategic document that would outline yearly targets.

Parameters of the service. The clinical team with UKCORE developed a plan of a patient's pathway through the hospital. It was then identified that the focus of the occupational therapy service was to support the clients' engagement in occupation in order to promote health and reduce or manage risk and offending behaviour. This is achieved through the Model of Human Occupation (MoHO). The service was outlined in terms of when the occupational therapy service would be offered, where it would be offered, what the content of the service would be, how the intervention would be graded. This collaboration developed a theory driven framework for the occupational therapy service.

R&D Strategic Document. This documentation needed to take into account what TSH occupational therapists were being asked to deliver in terms of governmental, institutional and professional priorities. Collaborative working synthesized these priorities into a workable document to support the change process. The document outlined the focus of the service, the challenges that face occupational therapy in developing its research base and an action plan outlining specifically the developments that were planned for the next 12 months. This document is used as a communication mechanism both for the wider institution and for occupational therapists who are all charged in delivering the change. The document is presented at hospital meetings and becomes part of the overall hospitals' strategic plans. Moreover, the strategic document allows for regular monitoring of progress through the change process.

(b) Managerial structures. Managerial structures were also identified as having important influence on change (Fitzgerald et al., 2003; McCluskey & Cusick, 2002). TSH already worked with their human resource department to develop job descriptions that explicitly identified research as part of all clinical posts and thereby legitimised research as an integral part of clinical life. This in and of itself was not enough to support the change to happen. The partnership took the information identified as the parameters of the service and integrated these within an integrated care pathway (Duncan & Moody, 2003).

Integrated Care Pathway (ICP). The integrated care pathway (ICP) outlines and documents clearly the key components of an individual's care within a given service. This provides a transparent set of guidelines around what service the occupational therapists should provide. These expectations are based on available evidence and include when an occupational therapy service should commence, what aspects of the client should be assessed, how the results of assessment are documented in the client's note, if the patient has reviewed the results of assessment. All of these are based within an expected timeframe (Duncan & Moody, 2003). This document is shared with other team members. The ICP is then reviewed by the hospitals clinical effectiveness department, to ascertain if these set evidence-based standards have been met. Statements can then be made as to how well occupational therapy is delivering evidence-based care.

Evidence-Based Assessment Protocols. Simultaneously evidence-based assessment protocols were developed. These are statements of clinical reasoning around the standard assessments that would be used at particular points in the patient journey. Groups of occupational therapists worked with academics within the partnership to select the appropriate evidenced-based assessments for clients at differing stages of their stay within the hospital (admission, treatment, and focused rehabilitation). These clinical and academic partnerships then tracked the patient journey through from admission to discharge to ensure there was enough information gathered to inform the "transitions" of the patient through the service. See Figure 2 for an example of a discharge assessment protocol. This protocol informs the decision making process around the transition of the patient from the hospital. Information is, therefore, needed about the patient's current ability to engage in everyday activity to know how much structure is needed in the new environment. Decisions were made that the Occupational Circumstances Interview and Rating Scale (OCAIRS) is a reliable and valid assessment that would provide an overview of the therapist's view of the client's current abilities. If the client was verbally cooperative and had sufficient insight an Occupational Self Assessment (OSA) would be encouraged as it provides the clients' view of their abilities and values. It was also determined that a detailed assessment of skill would be helpful for planning discharge. The Assessment of Motor and Process Skills and the Assessment of Communication and Interaction Skills were, therefore, chosen for this purpose. For those clients who were hoping to move towards work on discharge, the Work Role Interview was recommended. The assessments would be individually chosen from this range depending on the client's needs. This information would then be used to inform discharge planning.

Supervision Structures. Supervision structures were then examined to allow for evidence-based clinical responsibility to be supported on an individual basis. Regular supervision meetings were already part of the structure. The content of these meetings were developed to include active reflection on delivery of evidence-based practice. In addition to reflections on conceptualising cases through theory, cases are also discussed with reference to the most appropriate evidence based assessment choices. This allows staff to explore these issues with a mentor in privacy.

Leadership. Strong clinical leadership can be effective in supporting a change process (Locock et al., 2001; FoNS, 2001). It has

FIGURE 2. Discharge Protocol for Clients with No Positive Symptoms or Well Managed Positive Symptoms

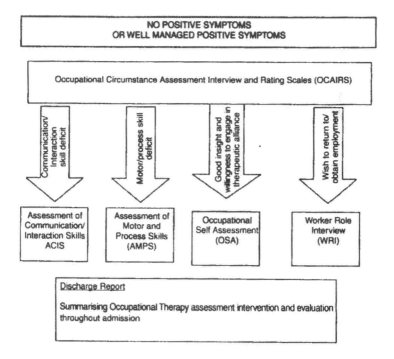

also been identified that it is important to develop clinical/academic career pathways, which define leadership roles (Scottish Executive, 2002; HEFEC, 2001). The TSH/UKCORE partnership has identified and created positions such as a Head Research Practitioner to provide leadership and act as a link person between the academics and clinicians. Their responsibility is to support the delivery of the R&D strategy and deliver expert evidence based, clinical practice. This post has ring-fenced time and is directly supported by UKCORE staff.

(c) Evidence-based development groups for staff. The partnership wanted to support clinicians as much as possible. It was identified in the literature that encouraging clinicians to work in small groups may help to maintain motivation and provide practical support (Conroy, 1997). All partners wanted to allow for consultation and engagement with the wider staff group routinely as part of the change process (Kaner et al., 2002). Working groups were, therefore, also set up to support the wider staff group to implement change. These groups meet routinely and are venues of sharing experiences and problem solving around barriers. They provide peer support. Any challenges that need further discussions are then taken to the steering group to access further support.

OUTCOMES OF SCHOLARSHIP OF PRACTICE

The outcomes of Scholarship of Practice include the delivery of evidence-based practice and the generation of evidence-based practice (see Figure 3).

Evidence of Delivering Evidence-Based Practice

The TSH/UKCORE partnership has successfully supported changes in practice. Practice changes have supported the use of evidence-based theory in practice. The changes have included the redevelopment of group work interventions, the focus of a staff on systematic implementation of evidence-based practice assessments through the integrated care pathway, completion of a robust research infra structure, development of a clinical research leader and clinical research career pathway, dissemination of good practice in national forums, delivery of evidence-based practice education, raised awareness of occupational therapists services within the health organization, and redesign of service provision.

FIGURE 3. Delivering and Generating Evidence-Based Practice

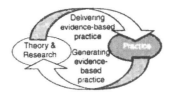

Practitioners Generating Evidence for Practice

Clinicians have contributed to the generation of theory and research through three international occupation focused outcome measures in the areas of vocational needs and adult disabilities. TSH practitioners were involved in ascertaining manuals for clinical utility, contributing to revision process of manuals, data collecting for reliability studies, clinical interpretation of statistical results and ongoing refinement of the assessments. This allowed the clinicians at TSH to input into a wider process of assessment development. This process allows for different perspectives to come together to build a scientific measure that has clinical utility. For example, academics bring knowledge around theory and statistics, practitioners bring knowledge about the practical realities of the clinical context and clinical experience, clients bring knowledge of their experience of services, managers bring their knowledge of what kinds of evidence they need to argue for more resources, and students bring their knowledge of what they need to develop into experienced practitioners. The process of both academia and practice contributing to the development of these assessment has led to clinically useful outcome measures being available for the profession (Parkinson et al., 2002; Deshpande et al., 2003; Braveman et al., 2004).

The State Hospital/UKCORE partnership will be leading a revision of the interest checklist and group work. The interest checklist will be comprehensively reviewed, incorporating the views of both clients and staff. This will be achieved through the use of consensus methodology (Murphy et al., 1998). After developing the content of the interest checklist using consensus methodology and revising its administration procedure, its reliability and validity will be tested using the international research network that has been developed in conjunction with UK

CORE and the University of Illinois, Chicago. Future research will focus on developing occupation-focused theory driven, evidence-based practice interventions. For example, at THS a theoretically driven group programme is being developed to support the delivery of occupational therapy within a robust group format (Forsyth et al., 2004).

CONCLUSION

This paper argues for the integration of knowledge generation and utilisation in occupational therapy. It is further argued that all stakeholders in occupational therapy should be involved in embedding evidence-based practice into the clinical context while simultaneously generating evidence for practice. The profession should build communities of "practice scholars" to support occupational therapy to move forward in an evidence-based world.

REFERENCES

Bennett, S., Tooth, L., McKenna, K., Rodger, S., Strong. J., Ziviani, J., Mickan. S., Gibson, L. (2003). *Perceptions of evidence-based practice: A survey of Australian occupational therapists. Australian Journal of Occupational Therapy.* 50, 13-22.

Braveman, B., Velozo, C., Kielhofner, G., Robson, M., Fisher. G., Forsyth. K. (2003). *User's Manual for the Worker Role Interview (WRI) Version 2.0.* The American Occupational Therapy Association. Bethesda.

Conroy, M. (1997). "Why are you doing that?" A project to look for evidence of efficacy within occupational therapy. *British Journal of Occupational Therapy,* 60, 487-490.

Creek, J., Llott, I. (2002). *Scoping study of occupational therapy research and development activity in Scotland, Northern Ireland and Wales: Executive Summary,* College of Occupational Therapists, London.

Deshpande, S., Kielhofner, G., Henriksson, C., Haglund, L., Olson, L., Forsyth, K., Kulkarni, S. (2003). *User's Manual for the Occupational Circumstances Assessment and Interview Rating Scale Version 2.0. (OCAIRS)* The American Occupational Therapy Association, Bethesda.

Duncan, E. A. S., Forsyth, K., Ashby, M., Summerfield-Mann. L. (2004). Occupational therapy service strategy: Promoting health. reducing risk and offending behaviour in everyday activity. The State Hospital. Carstairs.

Duncan, E. A. S., Moody, K. (2003). Integrated care pathways in mental health settings: An occupational therapy perspective. *The British Journal of Occupational Therapy.* Vol. 66 (10) pp. 473-478.

Fitzgerland, L., Ferlie, E., Hawkins, C. (2003). Innovations in healthcare: How does credible evidence influence professionals? *Health and Social Care in the Community* 11 (3) 219-228.

Forsyth, K., Duncan, E., McEwan, A., Summerfield Mann, L. (2004). Theoretically based group protocol, UK Centre for Outcomes Research and Education (UKCORE), London Foundation of Nursing Studies (2001). *Taking Action: Moving towards evidence-based practice*. London: FoNS.

Godfrey, A. (2000). Policy changes in the National Health Service: Implications and opportunities for occupational therapists, *British Journal of Occupational Therapy*, 63 (5): 218-224.

Grol, R. (1997). Beliefs and evidence in changing clinical practice. *British Medical Journal*, 315, 418-421.

HEFCE (2001). *Promoting research in nursing and the allied health professions*. Report to Task group 3.

Humphries, D., Littlejohns, P., Victor, C., O'Halloran, P., Peacock, J. (2000). Implementing Evidence-Based Practice: Factors that Influence the Use of Research Evidence by Occupational Therapists. *The British Journal of Occupational Therapy, 63 (11), 516-522.*

Kaner, E., Steven, A., Cassidy, P. (2002). Implementation of a model for service delivery and organisation in mental healthcare: A qualitative exploration of service provider views, *Health and Social Care in the Community*, 11 (6) 519-527.

Kielhofner, G. (2005). Scholarship and Practice: Bridging the divide. *American Journal of Occupational Therapy*.

Kielhofner, G., Hammel, J., Finlayson, M., Helfrich, C., Taylor, R. (2004). Documenting outcomes of occupational therapy. *American Journal of Occupational Therapy*, 58 (1), 15-23.

Locock, L., Dopson, S., Chamber, D., Gabbay, J. (2001). Understanding opinion leaders roles. *Social Science and Medicine* 53, 745-757.

McCluskey, A., Cusick, A. (2002). Strategies for introducing evidence-based practice and changing clinical behaviour: A managers toolbox. *Australian Occupational Therapy Journal* 49, 63-70.

Metcalf, C., Perry, S., Bannigan, K., Lewin, R. J. P., Wisher, Klaber, S., Moffatt, J. (2001). Barriers to Implementing the Evidence Base in Four NHS Therapies. *Physiotherapy*, 87, 8 433-441.

Murphy, M. K., Black, N. A., Lamping, D. L. (1998). Consensus development methods and their use in clinical guidelines development. *Health Technology Assessment* 1998; 2 (3).

NHS Centre for Reviews and Dissemination (1999). Effective Health Care: Getting evidence into practice, The Royal Society of Medicine Press, The University of York.

Parkinson, S., Forsyth, K., Kielhofner, G. (2002). *User's Manual for the Model of Human Occupation Screening Tool (MOHOST)* Version 1.0, UKCORE. London.

Scottish Executive (2002). *Building on Success: Future directions for the allied health professions in Scotland.*

Taylor, R.R., Hammel, J., Braveman, B. (2004). Developing and evaluating community-based services through participatory action research: Two case examples. *American Journal of Occupational Therapy, 58 (1),* 73-82.

Completing the Cycle of Scholarship of Practice: A Model for Dissemination and Utilization of Evidence-Based Interventions

Elizabeth Walker Peterson, MPH, OTR/L
Elaine McMahon, MS, RN
Marianne Farkas, ScD
Jonathan Howland, PhD

SUMMARY. The scholarship of practice stresses that knowledge should arise out of a dialogue and collaboration between scholars and practitioners. Bringing evidence back to practice completes the scholarship of practice cycle. This article describes a strategic approach to the process of knowledge dissemination and utilization and how that ap-

Elizabeth Walker Peterson is Clinical Associate Professor, Department of Occupational Therapy, University of Illinois at Chicago, 1919 West Taylor Street, MC 811, Chicago, IL 60612 (E-mail: epeterso@uic.edu). Elaine McMahon is Wellness Programs Manager, Partnership for Healthy Aging, 465 Congress Street, Suite 301, Portland, ME 04101 (E-mail: mcmahe@mmc.org). Marianne Farkas is Research Associate Professor, Sargent College of Health and Rehabilitation Sciences, and Director of Training, Center for Psychiatric Rehabilitation, Boston University, 940 Commonwealth Avenue West, Boston, MA 02215 (E-mail: mfarkas@bu.edu). Jonathan Howland is Professor, Boston University School of Public Health, 715 Albany Street, TW2, Boston, MA 02218 (E-mail: jhowl@bu.edu).

[Haworth co-indexing entry note]: "Completing the Cycle of Scholarship of Practice: A Model for Dissemination and Utilization of Evidence-Based Interventions." Walker Peterson, Elizabeth et al. Co-published simultaneously in *Occupational Therapy in Health Care* (The Haworth Press, Inc.) Vol. 19, No. 1/2, 2005, pp. 31-46; and: *The Scholarship of Practice: Academic-Practice Collaborations for Promoting Occupational Therapy* (ed: Patricia Crist, and Gary Kielhofner) The Haworth Press, Inc., 2005, pp. 31-46. Single or multiple copies of this article are available for a fee from The Haworth Document Delivery Service [1-800-HAWORTH, 9:00 a.m. - 5:00 p.m. (EST). E-mail address: docdelivery@haworthpress.com].

Available online at http://www.haworthpress.com/web/OTHC
doi:10.1300/J003v19n01_04

proach was used to increase knowledge and utilization of the *Matter of Balance* fear of falling intervention among occupational therapy practitioners. To illustrate how the approach supported clinicians' efforts to engage in evidence-based practice, the paper features a description of actions taken by a Maine-based health care system to successfully integrate *Matter of Balance* into its programming. Recommendations to policy makers, researchers and clinicians based on the authors' experiences with approach are presented. *[Article copies available for a fee from The Haworth Document Delivery Service: 1-800-HAWORTH. E-mail address: <docdelivery@haworthpress.com> Website: <http://www.HaworthPress.com>* © 2005 by The Haworth Press, Inc. All rights reserved.]*

KEYWORDS. Information dissemination and utilization, occupational therapy, fear of falling

INTRODUCTION

The scholarship of practice stresses that knowledge should arise out of a dialogue and collaboration between scholars and practitioners. While evidence-based knowledge generated in this way is likely to be usable to occupational therapists in practice, initial clinician-researcher collaboration does not assure adoption by other clinicians. The cycle of a scholarship of practice is completed when evidence is brought back to practice.

The goal of this paper is to inform the transfer of knowledge from research to practice arenas by describing a strategic approach to the process of knowledge dissemination and utilization. We will illustrate the process by describing (1) how it was used to disseminate an intervention to reduce fear of falling to occupational therapy clinicians, and (2) specific actions taken by a Maine-based health care system to integrate the intervention into its programming.

ORIGINS AND EVALUATION OF MATTER OF BALANCE

Fear of falling is a lasting concern about falling resulting in avoidance of activities. The fear was initially described as a consequence of a serious fall (Murphy & Isaacs, 1982; Nevitt, Cummings Kidd, & Black,

1989). As an occupational therapist working in acute care, home care, and outpatient settings, the first author recognized that concerns about falling were not limited to older adults who had actually experienced a fall. The first author collaborated with the fourth author to hypothesize consequences of fear of falling, such as compromised volition (i.e., lack of a sense of efficacy in avoiding falls), activity curtailment and retreat from valued activities and roles, deconditioning, and subsequent increased fall risk. Many of those hypothesized consequences were confirmed by subsequent research (Peterson et al., 1999; Murphy, Williams, & Gill, 2002; Howland et al., 1998; Tinetti & Powell, 1993; Cumming, Salkeld, Thomas, & Szonyi, 2000).

To explore fear of falling among a general sample of community-dwelling older adults, a cross-sectional study was undertaken to describe the prevalence, intensity and co-variates of fear of falling in that population (Walker & Howland, 1991). Findings from that paper provided early evidence that fear of falling is common and intense among older adults and were recognized by a team of researchers developing a proposal to establish a National Institute of Aging-funded Roybal Center for the Enhancement of Late-Life Function at Boston University. The first author was asked to work with that team to lead the development of an 8-session, group-based intervention (*Matter of Balance*). The research team determined that the primary outcome of the *Matter of Balance* (MOB) program would be to increase falls self-efficacy, in other words, a person's confidence in his or her ability to engage in daily activities without falling.

The interdisciplinary nature of the Boston University Roybal Center (BURC) was an important influence on the development of the MOB program. BURC researchers brought expertise in psychology, nursing, injury epidemiology and physical therapy that is reflected in the program. For example, the psychologist on the team used principles of cognitive behavioral theory to lead development of the conceptual model that served as the basis of the program (Lachman et al., 1997). The model recognizes self-efficacy, outcome expectations, and attributions (i.e., explanations one gives for outcomes) as important influences on an older adults' sense of control over the course and consequences of aging (Peterson, 2003). The MOB program applies principles of cognitive behavioral theory by using cognitive restructuring exercises to address volitional attitudes and beliefs about falls before focusing on behaviors associated with the reduction of modifiable risk factors (Peterson, 2003).

Occupational therapy literature and the first author's experiences as a clinician also informed development of the program in many ways. In addition to using traditional occupational therapy group process theory and content (Howe & Schwartzberg, 2001), the program recognizes social and physical environments as important enablers of function for older adults by helping seniors build social networks and mitigate fall hazards in the home. Activities designed to build skill in fall prevention and management (e.g., role-play exercises to build assertiveness, exercises to increase ability to safely get up from the floor) are used throughout the program. Additionally, MOB features a client-centered approach (Law, Baptiste, & Mills, 1995). For example, following "self-study" exercises resulting in an individualized assessment of fall risk, participants are asked to prioritize risk factors they want to address during the program. Problem-solving strategies used to mitigate fall risks are taught and applied to a number of different situations in order to teach participants how to generalize skills.

The program was evaluated in the late 1990s using a cluster randomized field trial that enrolled 434 residents of senior housing who were age 60 or older, and reported activity restrictions due to fear of falling (Tennstedt et al., 1998). The unit of randomization was the senior housing site. Forty sites were recruited for participation and pair-matched on the basis of number of units and percent of minority residents. Follow- up data collected at 12 months showed that participants who attended at least five of the eight sessions reported improved falls efficacy relative to baseline. These subjects were also more active than controls, without increasing their rate of falls (Tennstedt et al., 1998).

Demonstrating that fear of falling can be mitigated helped to make fear of falling clinically relevant. Recognizing the responsibilities of facilitating timely and effective dissemination of the evidence-based intervention, BURC researchers developed a conceptual framework intended to guide the dissemination and utilization process (Farkas, Jette, Tennstedt, Haley, & Quinn, 2003). The remainder of this paper describes that framework and how it was used to disseminate the MOB program. Although we illustrate the use of the framework using a single intervention, the process involved is relevant to dissemination and utilization of any evidence-based intervention.

THE CONCEPTUAL FRAMEWORK:
EXPOSURE, EXPERIENCE, EXPERTISE, EMBEDDING

The conceptual framework is an adaptation of categories first used to describe varying intensities of training methods (Cohen, 1985; Farkas & Anthony, 2001). It includes four strategies: *exposure, experience, expertise* and *embedding* which are operationalized in terms of the intended audience (i.e., consumers, practitioners, researchers). The framework also discriminates between knowledge dissemination, a fairly simple process of communicating new evidence (Rogers, 1983), and knowledge utilization which is a more complex process.

Exposure strategies are knowledge dissemination methods that focus on the goal of increased recipients' knowledge (Farkas et al., 2003). The choice of a specific *exposure* method or channel of communication depends largely upon the characteristics of the targeted user. While researchers tend to value information drawn from peer-reviewed journals and scientific conferences (Shepherd, 1982; Prohaska, Peters, & Warren, 2000), providers typically avoid research literature (Cohen, 1979; Farkas et al., 2003) and tend to seek out new information presented in an interactive format, such as roundtable discussions occurring at professional conferences (Burdine & McLeory, 1992). Thus, publications such as *OT Practice* that provide concise summaries of research findings and focus on implications for practice can be important exposure sources for occupational therapy practitioners.

Experience strategies focus on the goal of increased awareness and positive attitudes towards new knowledge. While *experience* strategies help the targeted user to "get ready" to use an innovation or new information (National Center for the Dissemination of Disability Research, 1996), *expertise* strategies are knowledge utilization methods that focus on the goal of increased competence (Farkas et al., 2003). Continuing education programs are often used by health care clinicians as mechanisms to build expertise in a given program or technique. Interactive activities (e.g., role-play exercises) and opportunities to share personal goals associated with the training are important aspects of such programs.

Embedding strategies are knowledge utilization methods designed to increase use of the new findings or innovations over time (Farkas et al., 2003). This need to institutionalize knowledge in daily practice has long been recognized as one of the most difficult aspects of knowledge utilization (Altman, 1995; Backer, Liberman, & Kuehnel, 1986; Goodman & Steckler, 1989; Mittlemark, Hunt, Heath, & Schmid, 1993; Rogers, 1983; Rosenheck, 2001). Although embedding strategies such as the use of peer support groups or Internet list serves can be targeted to consumers or practitioners, most embedding strategies are focused on program or system level administrators because these are the main agents of change and the maintenance of change (Farkas et al., 2003). Strategies can include organizational change techniques to help organizations develop structures that support the use of the information (Nemec, Forbess, Cohen, Farkas, Rogers, & Anthony, 1991; Rosenheck, 2001) or strategies that affect resources to make the changes sustain over time, such as funding (Altman, 1995). Additionally, rules, legislation and public policies sanction noncompliance and can alter norms and expectations about what is appropriate. While administrators and providers may be respectful of scientific evidence, their decisions about what to implement on a daily basis are shaped more by these types of power structures, ingrained routines and established resource configurations than by the scientific evidence (Rosenheck, 2001; Simon, 1997).

USING THE FOUR E'S:
APPLICATION OF THE FRAMEWORK
TO MATTER OF BALANCE

Dissemination Strategies

This paper focuses on MOB dissemination and utilization methods targeted to occupational therapy clinicians. For comparative purposes, Table 1 presents multiple target populations and associated exposure, experience, expertise and embedding methods.

Program Exposure Strategies Targeted
to Occupational Therapy Clinicians

The BURCELLF team recognized that the Roybal website was the most important vehicle supporting program exposure to the practice community and designed the website with practitioners in mind. To increase *information seeking* (Paisley, 1993), rather than simply information *transfer*, the web site allows visitors to make direct inquiries to the BURCELLF administrator as well as view downloadable clips from videos associated with the program. More traditional exposure methods targeted to practitioners include presentations at local, national, and international professional conferences, radio interviews, and printed media. Printed media was utilized in many formats including

TABLE 1. Examples of Exposure, Experience, Expertise, Embedding Strategies Associated with *Matter of Balance*

STRATEGY	Exposure	Experience	Expertise	Embedding
GOAL	Increased knowledge	Increased knowledge and positive attitudes	Increased competence	Increased utilization over time
Target Populations: • Researchers	*Examples:* Peer-reviewed articles (research methods detailed); seminars; Email; web based information	*Examples:* Mentorship	*Examples:* Facilitator manual; facilitator training programs	*Examples:* Ongoing availability of experts; ongoing research funding
• Occupational therapy clinicians • Occupational therapy administrators	Conferences; radio interviews; newsletters; newspapers; practice-focused articles; electronic user groups	Videos; program visits; discussions with clinician role-models who have successfully used the program	Facilitator manuals; facilitator training programs	Programmatic, systems level technical assistance; organizational development; on-going supervision and use of quality assurance mechanisms; advocacy; implementation-focused mailings to users
• Consumers	Popular media; Community lectures; Websites	Role Models (peers, video-based, described case examples)	Participant manual; program sessions	On-going support meetings; feedback tools

(adapted from Farkas, Jette et al., 2003).

practice-focused articles published in professional magazines (e.g., *OT Practice*), newsletters published by large organizations advocating for seniors (e.g., the American Society on Aging) and professional organizations (e.g., the American Occupational Therapy Association Home and Community Health Special Interest Section Quarterly). The dissemination effort gained momentum when the program received the 1998 American Public Health Association Archstone Foundation Award for Excellence in Program Innovation.

Newspaper reporters pay attention to what their colleagues at other newspapers are reporting. Consequently, exposure of MOB intensified after a few stories about fear of falling and the MOB program were printed in widely circulated newspapers. News stories about MOB have typically occurred in waves since dissemination efforts were launched. One wave of interest in the program began with a front-page story about fear of falling in the *New York Times* (Kleinfield, 2003) and peaked with publication of an article on fear of falling in *AARP Magazine* (Gandell, 2003) and National Public Radio's broadcast of a story on fear of falling (National Public Radio, 2003). MOB researchers have played a critical role in supporting development of stories about MOB by providing "the story" of their work in laymen's terms with emphasis on the personal cost of fear of falling for seniors. Reporters often asked researchers for the names of local occupational therapists delivering the program, and names of seniors who could provide "testimonials." Providing this kind of information, with permission, fostered the development of highly readable articles that led to more interest in MOB.

Program Experience Strategies Targeted
to Occupational Therapy Clinicians

Occupational therapy clinicians participating in conference workshops gained confidence in their ability to implement MOB by watching videos that featured clinician role models implementing the program, and seniors' positive response to the intervention. Clinicians seeking more information about the experience of implementing MOB were initially directed to the individuals who implemented the program during the randomized trial. As more occupational therapy practitioners gained experience in program implementation, BURCELLF research team members were able to direct questions to practitioners in the field. Whenever possible, occupational therapists were informed of other therapists in their area with program experience. In this way, a local network of experienced MOB providers could be formed. Program visits (i.e., observation of MOB sessions led by experienced therapists) also became important sources of experience for interested clinicians.

Program Expertise Strategies Targeted
to Occupational Therapy Clinicians

The 140-page *MOB Facilitator Training Manual* (Tennstedt, Peterson, Lachman, & Jette, 1998) was developed for clinicians delivering the program. The manual is intended to build program providers' expertise by describing objectives, materials and activities and timelines associated with each of the MOB sessions. The manual includes information describing where program resources (e.g., adaptive equipment, health education publications, home safety assessments, exercise equipment) can be obtained. Handouts in the manual are intended to be copied, and are print-ready for use by participants.

In response to the demand for MOB facilitator training that followed the APHA's recognition of the MOB program with the Archstone award, three BURCELLF research team members formed Boston Health Interventions (BHI), Inc. as a mechanism to offer continuing education courses. The 5-8 hour courses provided through BHI were designed to teach health care providers how to implement the MOB program, and primarily targeted occupational therapy practitioners. Since 1999, BHI has provided 20 trainings and has trained over 600 health care providers across the U.S. and in Europe, most of whom were occupational therapists. As a result of these trainings, occupational therapists in many states, including Massachusetts, Rhode Island, Illinois and Arizona have implemented MOB.

Program Embedding Strategies Targeted to Health Care Administrators and Occupational Therapy Clinicians

Strategies associated with embedding MOB can be categorized in two ways: those initiated by the BURCELLF, and those initiated by organizations and agencies external to the BURCELLF with a vested interest in delivering and sustaining the program. It is important to reiterate that many factors influence program embedding. The BURCELLF focused on factors it could influence. Specifically, the Roybal Center sustained interest of program users by creating and using specialized mailing lists to inform groups about updates on the program. Other factors, such as funding for community-based programming and manpower shortages limiting the number of practitioners available to work in a given location, were recognized as beyond the control of the BURCELLF. In order to illustrate embedding strategies used by an agency external to the BURCELLF, this paper will focus on actions taken by administrators of the Partnership for Healthy Aging (PFHA), a not-for-profit organization established by MaineHealth, an integrated health care delivery system. Context for that discussion is provided by a brief introduction to the PFHA and summary exposure and dissemination activities involving the PFHA that led to program embedding.

Case Study: The Partnership for Healthy Aging (PFHA)

PFHA was established by the Maine Medical Center (a research and teaching hospital), Community Health Services (a home health care organization), and the Southern Maine Agency on Aging. Additional support and resources are drawn from the University of Southern Maine. PFHA offers older adults and their families a comprehensive resource for health promotion, wellness, social services, family caregiver support, and service integration. By collaborating with organizations and resources for older adults throughout the community, PFHA is able to provide a continuum of care and services to help older adults maintain function and independence. The organization's program development is guided and supported by members of the Caregiver and Wellness Committees who offer a wide range of expertise.

Maine is a rural state with the third oldest population in the nation (Meyer, 2001). Recognizing the importance of prevention and wellness programs to older adults, PFHA has developed a tradition of seeking evidence-based programs that can be brought to Maine, field tested in the greater Portland area, and then disseminated throughout the MaineHealth system and the state through the Aging Network. MOB was the first healthy aging program sought by PFHA for dissemination.

PFHA administrators engaged in a variety of exposure, experience and expertise activities before beginning efforts to integrate MOB into existing programming. These activities are summarized in Table 2. Ultimately, the decision to implement MOB was supported by MaineHealth administrators because the program was a good match with the PHFA mission; the PFHA, MaineHealth, and the Maine Medical Center were willing to contribute financial resources toward the program (because

TABLE 2. PFHA Exposure, Experience and Expertise Activities

	Activities
Exposure	• Search BURCELLF website • Initiate conversations with BURCELLF administrator to learn about resources available to support program implementation
Experience	• Initiate conversations with BURCELLF researchers with direct experience delivering the program
Expertise	• Provide MOB facilitator training to PFHA clinicians

fall prevention was recognized as a high priority); and the PFHA had the health care expertise needed to implement the program.

PFHA administrators took a series of actions that made it possible to integrate MOB into PFHA programming. First, because a single staff person would not be able to facilitate the program more than once a year, the decision was made to enroll 9 health care providers in the first MOB facilitator training. Training multiple individuals provided inter-disciplinary expertise and allowed the PFHA-based MOB facilitators to support each other in program delivery. Occupational therapists, physical therapists, and nurses who voiced an interest in the program and had flexible work schedules participated in the MOB facilitator training. Second, in an effort to offer more classes, a "Master Trainer" was identified to teach additional facilitators throughout the MaineHealth system. Third, PFHA administrators supported staff involvement in outreach efforts. For example, presentations to community dwelling older adults were used as a mechanism to recruit MOB participants. These presentations were made to individuals and community groups (e.g., physicians, housing coordinators, churches, the City of Portland Parks & Recreation Department, the Osteoporosis Health Network Support Group). PFHA also wrote about MOB in its quarterly newsletter that is mailed to over 5000 people, and developed a MOB program brochure in partnership with the MaineHealth Learning Resource Center. Efforts to introduce MOB to the community were expanded when the Community Television Network produced a 4-part series on MOB for *Healthviews*, a health education program sponsored by MaineHealth that is aired on public access television. The series was initially aired four times in one week and has been repeated 16-20 times. From this series a 20-minute video providing an overview of MOB was developed. That video has been used repeatedly in facilitator trainings and to market MOB to seniors.

Use of process evaluation methods designed to improve program quality and participant retention represents a fourth embedding strategy. A participant satisfaction tool designed to gather quantitative and qualitiative data about program quality and facilitator effectiveness serves as a source for data regarding important program outcomes (i.e., comfort in talking to others about concerns about falls, confidence in increasing activity levels, plans to continue exercising). The tool has helped to alert program facilitators to the need for changes to the MOB. Specifically, changes made to the MOB exercise component resulted directly from satisfaction survey findings. Peer feedback mechanisms led to program changes (i.e., use of discussion instead of written exer-

cises, increased attention to cultural sensitivity) that improved participant retention when the program was provided to members of the
Native American Maliseet tribe.

Building partnerships with organizations sharing a commitment to
improving the health of the community was perhaps the most important
embedding strategy used by PFHA administrators. Partnering with
community agencies (i.e., recreation departments, senior centers, and
senior housing complexes) led to staff time and space donations, and allowed for integration of MOB into other programming systems. Creative
partnerships also led the PFHA to external funding for the MOB program
(provided by the Maine's Bureau of Elder and Adult Services, Southern
Maine Agency on Aging, and the Administration on Aging) and supported PFHA-led dissemination of MOB throughout the state of Maine.

PFHA's efforts to bring MOB to Maine have been greatly enhanced
by working closely with BURCELLF and BHI. The advice and support
offered by individuals from those institutions made it possible to adapt
MOB to meet community needs, while maintaining fidelity to the program as developed at the Roybal Center. The results of the collaborative
efforts between the PFHA, BHI, and the BURCELLF have been im-
pressive. In 2001, the National Council on the Aging selected MOB in
Maine as one of seven exemplary programs for senior centers and other
facilities as part of a landmark national survey of 628 community-based
programs. The Aging States Project recognized Maine for the dissemination of MOB, which was chosen as one of eight promising programs
in the country. In May 2003, the AoA acknowledged PFHA and BEAS
for dissemination of MOB, one of three exemplary best practices in
physical activity and aging. The Assistant Secretary of AoA featured
the program in the October 2003 edition of the *Journal of Physical Activity and Aging* in a guest editorial (Carbonell, 2003). News of these
awards and recognitions further exposed occupational therapy clinicians to MOB, opening the possibility for replication of the exposure,
experience, expertise and embedding cycle.

RECOMMENDATIONS

Over the past six years our dissemination and utilization activities
have generated a number of insights into ways practitioners can be supported in their efforts to access and use evidence in practice. The following recommendations regarding dissemination of evidence-based
programs are intended to support occupational therapy practitioners' efforts to initiate and sustain delivery of evidence-based services.

Policy. Our policy recommendations are two-fold. First, funding agencies should require a dissemination plan for all studies with practice implications. Such dissemination plans should be of high quality, invoking what is known about effective dissemination and utilization of information. Second, funding agencies should improve funding for dissemination and utilization efforts. Dissemination practices tend to be the least funded activity within research grants (Shepard, 1982).

Research. Our research recommendations focus on the composition of research teams. First, in concert with the scholarship of practice vision (Kielhofner, in press), we recommend the involvement of occupational therapy clinicians in research exploring occupational therapy practice issues. Involving clinicians as members of research teams has many benefits, from identification of clinically meaningful research questions to development of logistically feasible and practice-relevant interventions. Second, researchers should consider the dissemination benefits associated with the creation of interdisciplinary research teams. In our experience, use of interdisciplinary teams clearly supported dissemination across professions.

Practice. The transition from research to practice will be made easier if program under consideration is firmly based on theoretical models that are applicable to population served, and if the evidence-based outcomes associated with the program are well matched to the missions of agencies involved. Recently the APHA summarized data obtained by Archstone Award winners (including MOB researchers) and published a report that summarizes factors associated with evidence-based programs that have been successfully utilized by practitioners and sustained over time (Evashwick, Ory, & Smith, 2003). The lessons learned include the need to seek strong leadership, involve communities and key stakeholders, build on supporting organizational infrastructure, engage in active marketing, gather outcome data, seek seed money for start up funds, maintain shared organizational vision, and involve a university selectively (Evashwick et al., 2003). The lessons gleaned by following award-winning programs over time are highly relevant to occupational therapy clinicians and resonate with the PFHA experience.

CONCLUSION

As noted at the outset, the scholarship of practice involves a dialogue between practice and research. Part of that dialogue involved returning the results of research to practice. As noted by Kielhofner and Crist

(2005) too often research evidence does not make its way to practice. This means that researchers, among other things, have an obligation to return the evidence they generate to practitioners. This paper described and illustrated a conceptual framework that was successful in bringing an evidence-based intervention to practitioners. The conceptual framework for knowledge dissemination and utilization described in this paper expanded the range of dissemination efforts. As such, it was successful in enabling occupational therapists to incorporate an evidence-based intervention into their daily practice. Application of the framework of *exposure*, *experience*, *expertise*, and *embedding* to other research initiatives will help researchers take a more active role in dissemination/utilization efforts, increase clinicians' access to evidence-based programs, and ultimately increase the quality of the occupational therapy services delivered.

REFERENCES

Altman, D. (1995). Sustaining interventions in community systems: On the relationship between researchers and communities. *Health Psychology, 14*, 526-536.

Backer, T. E., Liberman, R. P., & Kuehnel, T. G. (1986). Dissemination and adoption of innovative psychosocial interventions. *Journal of Consulting and Clinical Psychology, 54*, 111-118.

Burdine, J., & McLeroy, K. (1992). Practitioner's use of theory: Examples from a workgroup. *Health Education Quarterly, 19*, 331-340.

Carbonell, J. G. (2003). Together we can increase physical activity among older adults. *Journal of Aging and Physical Activity, 11*, 427-432.

Cohen, H. L. (1979). The research readership and information source reliance of clinical psychologists. *Professional Psychology, 10*, 780-785.

Cumming, R. G., Salkeld, G., Thomas, M., & Szonyi, G. (2000). Prospective study of the impact of fear of falling on activities of daily living, SF-36 scores, and nursing home admission. *Journal of Gerontology: Medical Sciences, 55A*, 299-305.

Evashwick, C., Ory, M., & Smith, P. (2003). *Innovations in senior services: Highlights and lessons learned–A five-year review–1998-2002*. Long Beach. CA: Archstone Foundation.

Farkas, M., & Anthony, W. A. (2001). Overview of psychiatric rehabilitation education: Concepts of training and skill development. *Rehabilitation Education, 15*, 119-132.

Farkas, M., Jette, A., Tennstedt, S., Haley, S., & Quinn, V. (2003). Knowledge Dissemination and Utilization in Gerontology: An organizing framework. *The Gerontologist, 47, Special Issue I*, 47-56.

Gandell, C. (2003, July/August). Going steady. *AARP Magazine*, 68-73.

Goodman, R. M., & Steckler, A. (1989). A model for the institutionalization of health promotion programs. *Family and Community Health, 11*, 63-78.

Howe, M. C., & Schwartzberg, S. L. (2001). *A functional approach to group work in Occupational Therapy* (3rd ed.). Philadelphia: Lippincott, Williams & Wilkins.

Howland, J., Lachman, M. E., Peterson, E. W., Cote, J., Kasten, L., & Jette, A. (1998). Covariates of fear of falling and associated activity curtailment. *The Gerontologist, 38,* 549-555.

Kielhofner, G. & Crist, P. (Accepted) A Scholarship of Practice: Creating discourse between theory, research and practice. *Occupational Therapy in Health Care.*

Kielhofner, G. (2005). Scholarship and Practice: Bridging the Divide. *American Journal of Occupational Therapy.*

Kleinfield, N. R. (2003, March 5). For elderly, fear of falling is a risk in itself. *The New York Times,* pp. A1, A 25.

Lachman, M. A., Jette, A., Tennstedt, S., Howland, J., Harris, B. A., & Peterson, E. (1997). A cognitive-behavioural model for promoting physical exercise in older adults. *Journal of Psychology, Health and Medicine, 2,* 251-261.

Law, M., Baptiste, S., & Mills, J. (1995). Client-centered practice: What does it mean and does it make a difference? *Canadian Journal of Occupational Therapy, 62,* 250-257.

Meyer, J. (2001). Age: 2000-Census 2000 brief, pg. 4 Retrieved March 11, 2004, from http://www.census.gov/prod/2001pubs/c2kbr01-12.pdf

Mittlemark, M., Hunt, M., Heath, G., & Schmid, T. (1993). Realistic outcomes: Lessons from community-based research and demonstration programs for the prevention of cardiovascular disease. *Journal of Public Health Policy, 4,* 437-462.

Murphy, J. & Isaacs, B. (1982). The post-fall syndrome: A study of 36 elderly patients. *Gerontology, 28,* 265-270.

Murphy, S. L., Williams, C. S., & Gill, T. M. (2002). Characteristics associated with fear of falling and activity restriction among community-living older persons. *Journal of the American Geriatrics Society, 50,* 516-520.

Nemec, P. B., Forbess, R., Cohen, M. R., Farkas, M., Rogers, E. S., & Anthony, W. (1991). Effectiveness of technical assistance in the development of psychiatric rehabilitation programs. *The Journal of Mental Health Administration, 18,* 1-11.

Nevitt, M. C., Cummings, S. R., Kidd, S., Black, D. (1989). Risk factors for recurrent nonsynocopal falls: A prospective study. *Journal of the American Medical Association, 261,* 2663-2668.

Paisley, W. (1993). Knowledge utilization: The role of new communication technologies. *Journal of the American Society for Information Science, 44,* 222-234.

Peterson, E. (2003). Using cognitive behavioral strategies to reduce fear of falling: A matter of balance. *Journal of the American Society on Aging, XXVI (4),* 53-59.

Profile: Fear of falling lead elderly to inactivity. (2003, November 25.) Retrieved November 25, 2003 from http://www.npr.org

Prohaska, T. R., Peters, K. E., & Warren, J. S. (2000). Health behavior: From research to community practice. In G. Albrecht et al. (Eds.), The *handbook of social studies in health and medicine* (pp. 359-373). London: Sage Publications.

Rogers, E. M. (1995). The challenge: Lessons for guidelines from the diffusion of innovations. *Journal on Quality Improvement, 21,* 324-328.

Rosenheck, R. (2001). Organizational process: A missing link between research and practice. *Psychiatric Services, 52,* 1607-1612.

Sheperd, P. L. (1982). Theory to practice: The elusive marriage. *Gerontology & Geriatrics Education, 3,* 155-159.

Simon. H. (1997). *Administrative behavior: A study of decision-making processes in administrative organizations* (4th ed.). New York: Free Press.

Tennstedt, S., Howland, J., Lachman, M., Peterson, E. W., Kasten, L., & Jette, A. (1998). A randomized, controlled trial of a group intervention to reduce fear of falling and associated activity restriction in older adults. *Journal of Gerontology: Psychological Sciences, 53B*, 383-394.

Tennstedt. S., Peterson, E., Lachman. M., & Jette, A. (1998). *A Matter of Balance Facilitator Training Manual.* Boston University: Boston, MA.

Tinetti, M. E., & Powell, L. (1993). Fear of falling and low self-efficacy: A case of dependence in elderly persons. *Journal of Gerontology, 48,* 35-38.

Walker, J. E. & Howland, J. (1991). Falls and fear of falling among elderly persons living in the community: Occupational therapy interventions. *The American Journal of Occupational Therapy, 45,* 119-122.

A Model
of University-Community Partnerships
for Occupational Therapy Scholarship
and Practice

Yolanda Suarez-Balcazar, PhD
Joy Hammel, PhD, OTR/L, FAOTA
Christine Helfrich, PhD, OTR/L
Jennifer Thomas
Tom Wilson
Daphyne Head-Ball

SUMMARY. University-community partnerships are at the heart of community-based Occupational Therapy and the Scholarship of Practice that links practice with theory and research. In these partnerships, academicians, students, practitioners and staff from community organizations work in collaboration with a variety of community settings and programs, involving community leaders, agency staff, and/or members

Yolanda Suarez-Balcazar and Joy Hammel are both Associate Professors, Department of Occupational Therapy, University of Illinois at Chicago, 1919 West Taylor Street, MC-811, Chicago, IL 60612. Christine Helfrich is Assistant Professor, Department of Occupational Therapy, University of Illinois at Chicago. Jennifer Thomas and Tom Wilson are affiliated with Access Living, 614 W. Roosevelt Road, Chicago, IL 60607. Daphyne Head-Ball was Director of Transitional Housing at Family Rescue, Chicago, IL.

[Haworth co-indexing entry note]: "A Model of University-Community Partnerships for Occupational Therapy." Suarez-Balcazar et al. Co-published simultaneously in *Occupational Therapy in Health Care* (The Haworth Press, Inc.) Vol. 19, No. 1/2, 2005, pp. 47-70; and: *The Scholarship of Practice: Acudemic-Practice Collaborations for Promoting Occupational Therapy* (ed: Patricia Crist, and Gary Kielhofner) The Haworth Press, Inc., 2005, pp. 47-70. Single or multiple copies of this article are available for a fee from The Haworth Document Delivery Service [1-800-HAWORTH. 9:00 a.m. - 5:00 p.m. (EST). E-mail address: docdelivery@haworthpress.com].

Available online at http://www.haworthpress.com/web/OTHC
© 2005 by The Haworth Press, Inc. All rights reserved.
doi:10.1300/J003v19n01_05

of grassroots groups. This paper presents a framework of seven characteristics that are typical of successful partnership endeavors, such as
building a relationship based on trust and mutual respect. We illustrate
how this model can be used to promote praxis between theory, research
and practice with two examples of ongoing community partnerships that
involve an educational community practicum for all entry-level OT students. We also discuss the benefits and challenges of such partnership
and discuss the implications for community-based OT. *[Article copies
available for a fee from The Haworth Document Delivery Service: 1-800-
HAWORTH. E-mail address: <docdelivery@haworthpress.com> Website:
<http://www.HaworthPress.com> © 2005 by The Haworth Press, Inc. All rights
reserved.]*

KEYWORDS. Collaboration, partnerships, participatory research

In recent years, institutions of higher education have become more
interested in linking with community settings to develop partnerships to
examine ways that scientific knowledge and community experiential
knowledge can come together to address complex social problems. To
this regard, some institutions have expanded their service learning opportunities (see Carr, 2002; Greenberg, Howard, & Desmond, 2003),
while others have embraced what is called a scholarship of engagement
with communities, in which research is done in collaboration with community settings (e.g., Jackson & Reddick, 1999; Sanstad, Stall, Goldstein,
Everett, & Brousseaun, 1999). This engaged scholarship model has
been specifically applied to occupational therapy within the *Scholarship of Practice* framework that intertwines practice and research opportunities (Hammel, Finlayson, Kielhofner, Helfrich, & Peterson, 2002).
Authentic engagement with community organizations is essential to
furthering a *Scholarship of Practice* framework in occupational therapy
(Braveman, Helfrich, & Fisher, 2001). Embedding this engagement
within a required community practicum for entry-level OT students is
especially relevant to OT educators given the profession's long history
of "learning by doing." Most of these community settings involve agencies that provide social, health and consumer advocacy services to a variety of disadvantaged populations.

In OT-community partnerships, following a *Scholarship of Practice*
framework, the agenda is decided in collaboration with and is guided by
the needs of the community rather than the researcher or educator
(Bravemen, Helfrich, & Fisher, 2001) and the scholarship is designed to

result in action. This principle is consistent with Freire's (1970) praxis framework in which an ongoing interaction between reflection and action is achieved through a process of community and critical consciousness building *from within* the community. Freire's (1970) and Lewin's (1946) early work on action research laid the groundwork for Participatory Action Research (PAR). In PAR, community partners are involved in every step of the research, educational and practice process. The problem originates in the community and is defined, analyzed, and solved by the community (Balcazar, Keys, Kaplan, & Suarez-Balcazar, 1998; Selener, 1997). Within this approach, partners engage in joint reflection and analysis of needs and values of the community, collaborate in the research endeavors, and use findings to support social change efforts and support practice. Knowledge accumulation and theory building take place through participation in multiple attempts to change social systems (Argyris, Putnam, & Smith, 1985; Prilleltensky, 2001). The university-community partnerships model we proposed for OT *Scholarship and Practice* is then based on a PAR approach.

Truly collaborative university-community partnerships produce knowledge and outcomes that are significant and relevant to the community (Braveman et al., 2001; Suarez-Balcazar et al., 2004; Suarez-Balcazar, Harper, & Lewis, in press). In collaborations the scholarship and practice agenda is guided by the identified needs of the community setting or community. For the partnership to be successful, it needs to meet a need for the organization, which is likely to result in increased utilization of findings and social action (Panet-Raymond, 1992; Perkins & Wandersman, 1990; Selener, 1997).

University-community partnerships involve researchers and students working together with community leaders, service providers and consumers in a process in which constituents have an opportunity to shape and inform both practice and research, therefore improving programming and the quality of life for constituents. This paper proposes a framework of key principles and characteristics for developing and maintaining university-community partnerships that are consistent with the *Scholarship of Practice* framework and PAR. Based on a review of the literature on partnerships and our own collective experience, we developed a framework that includes three main process phases and a set of principles of authentic collaborative partnerships that are then illustrated within two different case studies. The *Scholarship of Practice* framework that we followed emphasizes strong relationships with community settings that reflect the real life issues of the community, and advance community-based OT research and practice (Hammel et al., 2002).

At the University of Illinois at Chicago, entry-level OT students take a community practicum in which they work within a community-based organization over the course of two semesters, placing students into a cognitive apprentice position (Hammel et al., 2002). Students are assigned to a community organization in which their faculty advisor has an ongoing research and educational relationship, and the advisor/faculty becomes the liaison between the students and the agency staff. For the most part, these community sites are agencies providing services to mostly low-income individuals and minority urban populations including people with disabilities, older adults, victims of domestic violence, low-income children and families from a community day care center, and people living with AIDS. What follows is a description of the key principles and characteristics of successful partnership endeavors.

DEVELOPING AND MAINTAINING PARTNERSHIPS FOR SCHOLARSHIP AND PRACTICE

Researchers from a variety of fields have proposed partnership models that vary from those that describe critical phases of collaborative research (e.g., Harper & Salina, 2000; Suarez-Balcazar & Orellana, 1999); to methodological strategies of Participatory Action Research (Balcazar, Keys, & Suarez-Balcazar, 2001; Taylor, Braveman, & Hammel, 2004); to characteristics of successful partnerships for research (Braveman et al., 2001; Suarez-Balcazar et al., 2004); to conceptual models of collaboration (e.g., Suarez-Balcazar et al., in press; Thompson, Story, & Butler, 2003). The proposed framework, adapted from Suarez-Balcazar et al. (2004) and Suarez-Balcazar et al. (in press) applies directly to Occupational Therapy Scholarship and Practice and provides a blueprint for OT researchers and practitioners. The framework includes three phases: pre-condition which includes building entry and competence; the process of building and maintaining the partnership; and outcomes of partnerships.

I. PRE-CONDITION: BUILDING ENTRY AND COMPETENCE

The first step in developing partnerships is gaining entry into the community agency and building competence in culturally understanding the community setting and its constituency. Initial contact can be established via existing connections, common interests, grant collaborations, and volunteering at the setting. Specific activities that facilitate this entry process include learning about the community agency, its programs, mission, and its population; visiting the agency and visiting with staff; touring the community; conducting participatory observations; and reviewing the literature on high priority issues for the agency and community that might inform practice. Once entry has been established, developing and sustaining the relationship over time is equally critical to show a long-term commitment to the community and engaged scholarship.

II. THE PROCESS OF BUILDING AND MAINTAINING THE PARTNERSHIP

Maintaining a collaborative relationship takes time and commitment to the partnership. The success and sustainability of partnership building involves the following seven principles: (a) developing a relationship based on trust and mutual respect, (b) establishing a reciprocal learning style, (c) developing open lines of communication, (d) maximizing resources, (e) using a multi-methods approach, (f) respecting diversity and building cultural competence, and (g) sharing accountability. Figure 1 illustrates the ongoing interaction of these principles. The principles are presented in no particular order as they are equally important and involve interactive processes that need to be attended to throughout the partnership.

a. Developing a Relationship Based on Trust and Mutual Respect

Establishing trust is facilitated by taking time to get to know the setting and the different stakeholders, agreeing on a common vision, setting expectations/ground rules, establishing common goals, and exchanging frameworks and ways of thinking about issues of importance. A common agenda and clarification of shared values needs to be pursued from the very beginning of the process. This first phase of developing trust is crucial to the success of any partnership and can be facilitated by fostering positive attitudes toward collaboration (Foster-Fishman, Berkowitz et al., 2001; Mattessich & Monsey, 1992).

From the beginning of the collaboration it is important to identify the community partner and key stakeholders within the organization with whom we will be working. However, partnerships call for flexibility in working with multiple layers of decision-makers (Mattessich & Monsey, 1992; Suarez-Balcazar et al., 2004). Community organizations have a

FIGURE 1. A Framework of University-Community Partnerships for Scholarship and Practice

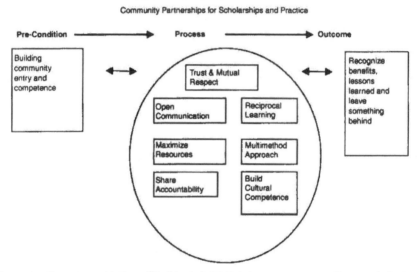

Adapted from Suarez-Balcazar, Y., Harper, W.G., & Lewis, R. (2005). An interactive and conceptual framework for building community-university partnerships for research and action. *Health Education and Behavior.*

number of stakeholders, from executive directors and staff members, to community constituents/members and community leaders. Given the constraints experienced by many agencies, such as staff turnover and work overload, our partner(s) might change throughout the partnership (Suarez-Balcazar, Orellana-Damacela, Portillo, Sharma, & Lanum, 2003). Therefore, it is important to establish a relationship with a range of community members and leaders and to share the OT scholarship and practice activities at the beginning of the partnership (Braveman et al., 2001). The scholarship and practice activities should be based on the needs of the community.

b. Developing Reciprocal Learning Opportunities

Each partner comes to the partnership ready to learn, as well as to guide. It is important for students as well as for faculty to enter the setting with an attitude of learning which sets in action a constant exchange of learning opportunities and flexible teacher-learner roles for all. Collaborative partnerships for OT research and practice recognize that there is knowledge in both the university and the community. The coming together of these types of knowledge challenges and eliminates false boundaries that occur when the knowledge solely resides in academia or the community. This interactive building of knowledge is congruent with a PAR approach. Unfortunately, community members' knowledge is often devalued by an illusion of superiority of academic expertise. Within a PAR and *Scholarship of Practice* framework, experiential knowledge and academic knowledge complement each other (Jason et al., 2004).

c. Establishing Open Lines of Communication

Establishing a good communication system is at the heart of authentic partnerships. This process focuses on what is communicated, how it is communicated, and the communication style and language used. Partnership goals, expected roles and outcomes are agreed upon early in the process (Connors & Seifer, 2000; Panet-Raymond, 1992). Given the complex nature of partnerships, goals and expectations may change throughout the process, and they need to be openly discussed and negotiated using formal and informal channels of communication. Being sensitive to the communication mode and style of the setting may imply using modes of communication that work for the setting, including formal memos, regularly scheduled meetings, e-mail messages, phone calls, and one-on-one visits (Suarez-Balcazar et al., 2005).

For a relationship to be successful, it is essential to establish open and frequent communication by providing updates, discussing issues openly, and sharing all information with one another as well as the broader community membership (Mattessich & Monsey, 1992). In the case of site supervisors working with students, it is important to establish regular ways of communicating such as weekly one-on-one meetings or emails in order to discuss how the partnership is unfolding, to quickly identify any issues and to strategize how to address them, and to sustain trust.

University partners will also be most successful at developing and sustaining an authentic relationship when using a non-hierarchical communication style (Harper et al., 2004; Suarez et al., 2004). This also means avoiding using academic language and jargon to impress the community. Often communities have been treated in condescending and paternalistic ways that impede a trustful relationship and tend to build resentment towards the university (Gills, Butler, Rose & Bivens, 2001).

d. Maximizing Resources

Each of the partners brings into the relationship a set of resources and strengths that need to be recognized and valued (Connors & Seifer, 2000; Mattessich & Monsey, 1992). Most typically, faculty and students bring access to resources (e.g., grant funding), knowledge of research design and methods and access to evidence-based literature sources, theoretical knowledge of the OT profession, and practical information of OT strategies and practice models. Our community partners bring knowledge of the specific area or population of interest, experiential information of the issues involved, and awareness of the cultural and contextual characteristics of the setting and community where they work/live (Braveman et al., 2001; Suarez-Balcazar, Muñoz & Fisher, in press). While the community might teach students and faculty about issues relevant to the community, we might teach them about the OT profession. It is not uncommon to find that few people outside of the OT profession know what OT scholarship and practice is. In many cases, agency staff also brings knowledge of research and theories from outside the OT profession that are likely to enrich OTs.

Our community partners play a critical role in enhancing the cultural competence of OT students by exposing them to urban populations and urban issues and teaching us about the issues they face (Suarez-Balcazar, Muñoz & Fisher, in press). For the most part, our entry level students have little experience working with marginalized populations, such as people with disabilities, victims of domestic violence, low-income minorities and people living with AIDS.

Resources such as time and space have a different meaning for both settings. Timeframes for researchers are based on the academic calendar and funding cycles, while the organization or community setting might be on a different timeline influenced by events like funding cycles, fund raising, upcoming events or social action initiatives, and the local school calendar (if they serve children). These resources need to be recognized and taken into consideration when scheduling scholarship or practice activities.

Resources might be perceived differently both in academia and the community. For instance, not all members of a community organization may have their own individual computer or access to the Internet, e-mail, etc. Grant funding may allow for some flexibility and the opportunity to cover research related expenses incurred by the partners; however, this only occurs if planned in advance into the grant by involving partners in the grant writing process. Additionally, for many people with disabilities, resources to support accommodations such as transportation, personal assistance, interpreting, and captioning are often critical to support their active participation. It is important to note that communities receive very little funding, if any, for research activities and that they may perceive research as a low priority. It is incumbent upon researchers and educators from universities to make a direct link between research, education practice so that the needs of the community are considered and the relationship yields mutual benefits.

e. Using a Multi-Method Approach to Scholarship and Practice

Both qualitative and quantitative strategies complement each other and provide the research and practicum agenda with multiple levels of analysis. Using multiple methodologies also enables the partners to obtain information on an ongoing basis and remain invested, as they often are able to use the evidence gained in their own action initiatives. At the same time that quantitative methodologies have enjoyed a long history in some basic and health sciences, qualitative methods have had a long history in the social sciences (Stewart, 2000). Qualitative methodologies with community agencies have been documented as being more sensitive and culturally relevant with diverse populations and disadvantaged communities (Suarez-Balcazar et al., 2003). Furthermore, site staff and supervisors might bring experience in using methods such as focus groups/listening sessions, interviews, participant observation, open-ended interviews, public forums/town halls and listening sessions. These strategies are likely to establish trust and rapport with participants (Tandom, Azelton, & Kelly, 1998). At the same time, quantitative findings may be valuable in equally influencing policy or systems change. Therefore, multiple methods that fit the needs of the community as well as inform the issues and action initiatives are recommended.

f. Respect Diversity and Build Cultural Competence

Velde and Wittman (2001) argued that OT researchers and students, as well as health care professionals in general, need to develop cultural competence to work in diverse communities. They assert that researchers and practitioners need certain knowledge, attitudes and skills related to diversity and multi-culturalism and need to learn about the population of interest before gaining entry into the setting. We have also found that after students have done some research learning about the population of interest and then experienced immersion into the setting that they find the experience enlightening and enriching.

For the most part, diversity is a characteristic of these partnerships and respecting and celebrating diversity becomes essential to the relationship and to building cultural competence (Nelson et al., 2001; Suarez-Balcazar, Durlak, & Smith, 1994; Suarez-Balcazar, Muñoz, & Fisher, in press; Velde & Wittman, 2001). Strategies that facilitate the process include learning about the community and its population in advance of and throughout the partnership process, learning about the culture and ethnic background represented by the population served by the agency via direct experience and time with this community, and reflecting on ones values, race and ethnic experiences and stereotypes that one might hold about a social group and the diversity of members within it. It is important to reflect on the values and ideas one might have about specific groups who are different from oneself (Suarez-Balcazar, Muñoz, & Fisher, in press).

Forming a diverse research team usually helps the partnership, but is no guarantee for success. We need to keep in mind that the typical OT student is a Caucasian, young female (Velde & Wittman, 2001). Therefore, we as faculty need to enhance our efforts in recruiting minority students into the profession, particularly people from the very communities with which we partner. Furthermore, we need to plan educational experiences designed to promote cultural competence in OT students, educators and researchers (Suarez-Balcazar, Muñoz & Fisher, 2000).

Specific skills that result from developing cultural competence include identifying the importance of culture and diversity, assessing cross-cultural relations, being vigilant towards the dynamics that result from cultural differences, being aware of one's beliefs and biases toward others, and adapting services, research endeavors and practice to meet the needs of diverse populations as defined from within those communities (Cross, Bazron, Dennis, & Isaacs, 1989; Suarez-Balcazar, Muñoz & Fisher, in press).

g. Sharing Accountability

Equally sharing the credit for accomplishments and successes is important to the maintenance of the partnership over time as it validates everyone's efforts and contributions (Blake & Moore, 2000). This might be done by writing the report in collaboration with the group, distributing publicity about the partnership within the academic institution and community, sharing responsibility for problems, misunderstandings and conflicts that may happen throughout the process, co-chairing control of the partnership's project, and importantly, acknowledging community partners in all information disseminated. This also includes targeting dissemination within the community through local resources like newsletters and websites versus only disseminating the information within academic, professional or research venues.

III. OUTCOMES AND IMPACT

If universities strategize in collaboration with the community, partnerships can result in multiple benefits for everyone involved. For truly collaborative partnerships under PAR and a *Scholarship of Practice* framework, the benefits to the agency and the community they represent need to be concrete and real. It is important to recognize that many community settings have a long history of being used by academic units and are often weary and reluctant to participate in future partnerships.

Recognizing Benefits, Lessons Learned, and Leaving Something Behind

Overall, partnerships bring in a number of benefits to both the university and the community. Community sites participating in partnerships may experience increased capacity, participation in funded grants, completion of tangible products as a result of the practicum, and direct benefits to participants such as new services/programs. Other benefits include shared ownership over products and strategies developed, development of new and shared knowledge, and adoption of innovations developed.

Some of the specific benefits for the university include: opportunities to advance scholarship activities, continued support for grant writing and grant funding, practicum experience for students, capacity building for faculty and students in enhancing cultural competence, increasing knowledge of diverse populations and knowledge of specific areas of research, and opportunities to engage in learning by doing.

University-community partnerships are not without their own challenges and lessons learned. These have been discussed extensively in the literature (e.g., Connors & Seifer, 2001; Mattessich & Monsey, 1992; Riger, 2001; Suarez-Balcazar et al., 2004). Some of these challenges include managing conflicts of interest, and different perspectives, sustaining activities after termination of funding, changing roles and redefining boundaries, developing common ground, managing different schedules, and different sets of pressures for all involved. Partnerships call for flexibility and a high level of tolerance given the complexity of collaborative endeavors. We need to acknowledge these challenges up front, openly discuss them, and strategize how to address them throughout the partnership.

The following case studies illustrate the principles of community partnership previously presented and some of the lessons learned, challenges faced, and strategies used to promote sustainable partnerships that cut across and inform research, education and practice.

TWO EXEMPLARS: SCHOLARSHIP OF PRACTICE AT WORK

Partnering and Promoting Praxis with a Center
for Independent Living Center

The first case study focuses on strategies and lessons learned related to building and sustaining a collaborative partnership between a university-based OT program and a Center for Independent Living (CIL). Three processes are examined: gaining entry and developing trust, developing cultural awareness, and using reciprocal learning and multiple methods. In this case, the "community" represents the disability community as a social or minority group. Since the goal of the UIC partnership with Access Living (AL), a regional Center for Independent Living, is to expose and immerse occupational therapy students into the disability experience from within that community, and the goal of Access Living is to promote activism and social justice within the disability community, using praxis as a framework is critical to promote an authentic collaboration to mutually inform theory, research and practice, both for the disability activism and occupational therapy communities. The primary faculty liaison, Joy Hammel, collaborated with AL across educational, research and practice activities to facilitate engaged scholarship (Hammel et al., 2002), and, in the process learning many lessons about community partnering.

Description of the Community Partner. Access Living (AL) is a Center for Independent Living (CIL) that is directed, majority led, and operated by people with disabilities, representing the Chicago urban community and approximately 26,000 constituents with disabilities. Its mission is to "provide services that promote the independence and the inclusion of people with disabilities in every aspect of community life. AL follows the independent living philosophy that calls for community-based, consumer-controlled service and advocacy programs that emphasize a cross-disability and self-help approach. Access Living recognizes the innate rights, abilities, needs and diversity of people with disabilities, works toward their integration into community life and serves as an agent of social change" (Access Living, 2004).

Establishing Entry, Rapport, Trust and Respect. Activities for entering AL included:

1. Creating an early relationship and line of communication between the faculty liaison and AL. Initial meetings allowed for a "testing out" period, in which AL staff challenged the liaison to discuss motivations for collaboration and to see if she had done her homework in understanding their community. As a potential partner, AL was clear that they did not want a relationship in which a medical model is imposed, in which they supported UIC but AL constituents did not directly benefit, or a short term relationship primarily to educate OT students. Instead, they requested social learning in which students and AL staff/ constituents learned from each other and AL staff were recognized as mentors, activities are prioritized to reflect those with the greatest long term impact for AL constituents; and, a long term relationship would be sustained.

2. Honing in and establishing a close working relationship with two specific programs within AL: the deinstitutionalization and personal assistance programs. These two programs represented the best opportunities for students to explore the disability experience at the individual, social group and social justice levels. By choosing specific programs, we were also able to solidify a close relationship with key program staff.

3. Inviting AL staff and disability studies scholars to present to UIC faculty and students on their philosophy, current systems change initiatives, and the intersects of activism and scholarship, providing a dialogue beyond the community practicum.

4. Collaborating on pilot research grants to examine community living and participation as framed by disabled constituents and to collect evidence for future research. This then led to many joint research projects, including a federal grant to create and evaluate a Social Action Group program to support people with disabilities in moving out of nursing homes to the community.

Promoting Cultural Competence. A critical area for the partnership focused on developing a cultural awareness of disability amongst students and researchers alike. To promote praxis, it is critical that partners know about each other's history, vision, mission, and ideologies. Importantly, this includes spending time learning about CILs as an organization and about disabled people as a minority group rather than imposing professional ideologies about disability "from outside" or "over" the community. We need to understand the cultural context of a CIL, as well as the cultural diversity and differences within its constituency base. Following is a discussion of targeted areas of cultural immersion and praxis.

Comparing CIL History and Theory with Occupational Therapy. The history and guiding theoretical framework of CILs focuses at the level of the social group. The Social Model of Disability (Oliver, 1996; Linton, 1998), and the related Minority Group Model (Longmore, 1995), view disabled people as a minority social group, in the same way other minority groups are constructed by race, ethnicity, age, gender, and sexual identity. Disability is framed as difference that in itself is neutral. Disability takes on a negative construction when barriers are imposed upon disabled people by society, such as lack of access to affordable and accessible housing, transportation, employment, school, and social opportunities. These inequities result in oppression of disabled people as a social group, and can result in alienation of this group and individuals within it when societal barriers affect participation and power (Charlton, 1998).

A Minority Group framing focuses on the building of critical consciousness and power *within* a social group (Charlton, 1998; Friere, 1970; Young, 1990). The diversity and difference of disabled people are acknowledged, respected and celebrated, rather than viewed as something to overcome or normalize as is often the case within a medical model approach. Similar to Black Pride and Gay Pride, the disability community as a minority group is working to reframe Disability from an overwhelmingly negative conceptualization to one of strength and collective consciousness. Thus, CIL philosophy is based upon sociological theory bases of materialism, social constructionism, feminism, race and minority group theory, and social justice.

Whereas CILs focus at the sociological level, occupational therapy practice and much of its research focus primarily on the level of the individual as he/she engages in occupations in his/her immediate context (social & physical), corresponding to an ecological, systems or social psychological theory base. Although the "environment," and its role as an influencing factor, is shared between CILs and OT, the two differ in their level of focus, and ergo, their practices. These differences can be viewed as critical dividing gaps, or as key points of praxis over which OT and CILs can dialogue, inform each other, and conceptualize new and innovative practice. Following are several examples of how this dialogue was used to promote this praxis.

What Is Disability and What Is Independence? Naming and Framing. As discussed previously, CILs frame disability as difference that can be constructed negatively or positively depending on the context and issues of power. CILs view people with disabilities as constituents and citizens within a social minority group, and within the society. Given a strong tie to rehabilitation framings of disability, occupational therapists view individuals with disabilities at the level of the patient, client or consumer of services. Disability has been framed as a negative dysfunction or deficit within the individual, or as a functional performance problem. Within a rehabilitative functional approach, independence is constructed as the physical and cognitive ability to perform everyday activities by oneself in a safe, timely and socially appropriate manner. CILs instead view independence as an issue of freedom: the freedom to do what you want to do, when, where and with whom you want to do it; as choice; as power over life decisions; and as control over everyday life and resources to support it.

Promoting Praxis on Disability and Independence. We used the community partnership with AL to expose students and researchers to alternative framings of disability and independence. Students met with disability activists who explained the history of the disability movement and societal barriers that continue to oppress. They read writings and watched videos that highlighted the experiences of disabled people and the barriers they have faced related to housing, transportation, and personal assistance (see books such as Charlton, 1998; Longmore, 2003; and Longmore & Umansky, 2001 for scholarship from within the disability community). They went with staff to meet disabled people, including people living in nursing homes or in the community on subsidized incomes of $540/month, witnessing first hand how oppression affects their control and choice, while at the same time coming to respect and recognize their resiliency and strengths as individuals and the collective power of the disability activism community.

CIL staff also highlighted how safety and risk are viewed differently. They strongly assert a right to make choices and therefore take "risks with dignity" in everyday life, viewing personal security and safety as a human rights issue (e.g., the right to live in a situation where one is not abused, violated or neglected). This is in comparison to a therapist's focus on whether a person is deemed to be safe and competent to live on one's own based on physical and cognitive function. These opportunities for social learning challenged students to critically analyze their professional conceptions of disability and independence, and to reflect on ways they, as practitioners, could highlight interdependence, access to support, freedom of choice, and human rights issues in their practice. In turn, OT students were able to offer a number of strategies, such as environmental adaptations, as tools to promote freedom and control, and to join the social action fight with AL to promote equitable access to these resources.

What Is Empowerment? Naming and Framing. Another key area of praxis occurred related to the empowerment. Within rehabilitation, empowerment is viewed at the level of individual control, power and choice. The focus is upon self-advocacy, or the ability to identify and advocate for one's needs and resources to support those needs. CILs fully support the concept of self-advocacy, and often focus their programming on working with constituents so they can access information, become informed self-advocates, and direct their own planning. However, CILs also acknowledge that individual advocacy by itself will not overcome the societal barriers or oppression that exist (Charlton, 1998). CILs also support critical consciousness building, including the creation and sharing of the history, narratives, art and culture of disabled people for disabled people. Thus empowerment goes beyond individual self-advocacy to collective activism and community building *"from within"* (Friere, 1970; Longmore, 1995).

Praxis on Empowerment. Within the community partnership, OT students become part of the individual self-advocacy efforts that CIL staff facilitated during peer counseling and small group programming, coming to recognize the power of a peer mentoring approach. They also participated in collective activism initiatives in the community. Students repeatedly discussed that participating in social action events, such as a sit-in or a rally to protest existing oppression, were the most powerful activities in transforming their conceptions of disability. Through these, they witnessed the collective strength and power of this disability community, something that is not seen in individual therapy sessions. Similarly, reading the narratives and watching the videos and performance art produced by disabled artists, writers, and scholars was also transformative in recognizing the consciousness of this group. In turn, students linked disabled constituents with information technology (IT) to socially network and explore the disability community and the arts.

While students were learning via this community practicum, the UIC students and faculty collaborated with AL to also begin a series of research projects that furthered this reframing of disability, independence and empowerment. Research included qualitative exploration of the disability experience in the urban community, examination of the societal barriers, and systems change to address issues of power and control. Practicum students became a part of this research while on site at AL; several completed Master's projects and theses that contributed to this line of inquiry; and praxis between activism and scholarship was sustained.

Summary. This case study illustrates how a community partnership with a CIL not only fostered learning about the disability experience *from within,* but also facilitated praxis and the critical dialectic between activism and reflection that can transform how students practice as occupational therapists as well as the scholarship of OTs. This quote from one of our partners illustrates how she views how this praxis can be transferred to the everyday practice of OTs: "As a person with a disability I believe it important for an OT to be seen as an ally for the person with the disability and to empower the person to believe in themselves and not see disability as a 'negative' occurrence in their life, but rather to help the person to gain the skills and to access the supports to live decently. As a 28-year-old woman with Cerebral Palsy who has had CP since birth, I live daily with the reminders of how an OT has been my ALLY to foster my independence and my freedom of choice. During these OT sessions, we don't have to do a physical task like dressing, as much as to brainstorm and strategize how to manage, like how can we mount baby carriers on my wheelchair so that I can transport my babies on my wheelchair."

Building a Relationship with a Domestic Violence Community Agency

The following case illustrates how (1) scholarship and practice partnership is based on the needs of the community, (2) developing reciprocal learning opportunities and maximizing resources, and (3) establishing open lines of communication are essential features of community collaboration. The relationship between the University of Illinois at Chicago (UIC) and Family Rescue began in 1993 when UIC was subcontracted to conduct an ethnographic program evaluation of a Head Start demonstration project funded by the Department of Human Services (Beer & Helfrich, 1996). That beginning placed the university in the position of being an outside expert, reviewing the organization's performance, and influencing the continued funding of their Head Start program.

Throughout the years, the university and community have developed and established a strong and multifaceted partnership, based on mutual respect and focusing on benefits.

Community Partner Description. Family Rescue is the largest comprehensive domestic violence agency in the state of Illinois providing emergency shelter, transitional housing and day care, court and legal services and community outreach. Their comprehensive response to domestic violence includes the provision of direct services to survivors and their families as well as systemic advocacy and community education. Women and children served by the agency are primarily low income, minority residents of the Chicago area. Services provided include crises management, legal advocacy, housing, and counseling. Life skills services are delivered through case management.

Scholarship and Practice Partnership Is Based on the Needs of the Community. Over the course of their ten-year partnership, individuals' roles at the university and the agency have shifted, transforming both the nature and focus of their relationship. As noted above, the relationship began with the university in the position of "outside evaluator." Based on the PAR approach used to conduct the evaluation, the researcher began developing a collaborative relationship learning the values, needs and priorities of the agency. Through that process, the third author responded to those needs by (1) designing her dissertation to further understand the experiences of women living in transitional housing (Helfrich, 1997), (2) creating OT fieldwork experiences during the summer to develop programs with the school aged children (Walens, Helfrich, Aviles, & Horita, 2000), (3) creating community practicum experiences in the Before and After School Program and the Transitional Housing Program to address life skills and (4) collaborating with the agency on grants designed to create allied health services with underserved communities and life skill intervention outcome studies. These collaborations resulted in practical learning experiences for students and raised community based research questions, which were subsequently addressed by the university partner through grants and thesis.

Developing Reciprocal Learning Opportunities and Maximizing Resources. Each subsequent collaboration has fostered a deeper partnership with the community where graduate students complete projects and thesis designed to meet program needs and research interests of the agency and where community partners participate in graduate classes as experts, mentor practicum and fieldwork students and serve on grant and curriculum advisory boards. The community partner has provided access to staff and clients throughout the agency for a variety of research studies and masters projects and mentored both the faculty member and her students to learn about the needs, culture, politics, concerns and values of the domestic violence and homeless communities. The interpersonal dynamics of domestic violence and the experiences that women endure while in an abusive relationship, when they leave the relationship and go to a shelter impact their ability to trust outsiders and health care providers in particular as they strive to maintain safety for themselves. Many of the women have encountered child protection services during their abuse and are reticent to sign consent forms for their children to participate in services with the OT students because they fear the child's records might be subpoenaed in court. Understanding these concerns has modified documentation procedures such as not using last names and only sharing assessment results verbally with parents and teachers rather than placing them in the child's folder. In return, the faculty member and OT students have brought their knowledge of activity analyses, life skills and program evaluation to address the unmet needs of the agency. The products that students have created such as group protocols and client satisfaction surveys have been institutionalized within the setting and adapted for more general use within the entire agency. For example, at the transitional housing program, the program director asked the students to develop and administer a client satisfaction survey to help the staff understand why clients did not feel comfortable communicating around issues of dissatisfaction. That same survey was modified and is now being used by the board of directors to evaluate client satisfaction throughout the agency. The resources that each partner has contributed allowed for learning and products to be created that neither one could have done without the other.

Open Lines of Communication. Throughout the partnership, the most essential factor has been to maintain open lines of communication based on mutual respect. The collaborative activities that students engage in take place with a diverse group of agency staff at several different physical sites thus complicating communication. In addition to the variety of staff with whom each student must communicate, the agency must also adjust to communicating with different students as they rotate through the OT program. This range of participants creates an environment that can be ripe for miscommunication and misunderstanding, unless both partners are vigilant about maintaining frequent clear and open communication. At the start of each new project, the partners meet face to face at the agency to clarify expectations and communication lines for that specific project. During project implementation, the faculty member checks in periodically with phone calls to the agency to provide a space to discuss any new issues or concerns; however, both partners have committed to calling the other at any point to clarify misunderstandings as they arise to ensure early clarification and problem solving. This commitment to good communication further enhances mutual respect and trust between the partners.

Summary. This case illustrates the complexity of a long, diverse collaboration between the university and a community partner. Over time, the collaboration and individual roles of the partners have changed and been negotiated to meet both individual and institutional needs. The diversity of collaborations has allowed the praxis between scholarship and practice to occur. Each learning and research opportunity informed others and led to additional projects being created. While the list of ongoing collaborative opportunities is endless, the success of anyone of them is dependent on mutual respect and mutual benefit to both partners.

DISCUSSION

University-community partnerships within a framework of *Scholarship of Practice* can become a catalyst for social change and can serve as a mechanism to improve services, and programs concerning minority communities and/or individuals who share a common predicament such as having a disability. Researchers and practitioners can become agents of social change when the research and practice activities within community settings are done in collaboration with staff and constituents and have the potential to be acted upon, resulting in direct benefits for consumers, and when research informs practice and practice informs research. Research and practicum experiences might be used to support the creation of new programs, improve existing services, and to support changes in policy. By working in collaboration and partnership with community members and leaders, researchers can join partners in disseminating reports, presenting findings to decision makers, the board of directors, and the community itself.

University-community partnerships are not without their challenges, but the many benefits and rewards maintain our involvement. We need to be ready to manage opposition and conflicts of interest. Often the substance and style of collaborative action research challenges the *status quo* in academic circles. While this is part of its appeal and value, one might expect questioning and discouragement from traditional researchers. Just as community leaders challenge elected officials or confront community institutions to bring about social change, change agents inside academia need to engage in long-term organizing to win support and neutralize internal opposition to community-university partnerships research.

In all, university-community partnerships are at the heart of community-based OT scholarship and practice. They provide an opportunity for academic and community partners to learn from one another, to address issues of relevance to the community of interest and to engage with the community in the ongoing praxis of reflection and action. University-community partnerships bring benefits for all involved. By working together, faculty, students and community members increase their skills and enhance their ability to study, understand and address issues that matter to our communities.

REFERENCES

Access Living (2004). *Access Living: Center for Service, Advocacy, and Social Change for People with Disabilities: Mission Statement.* Retrieved March 15, 2004, from *http://www.accessliving.org/*.

Argyris, C., Putnam, R., & Smith, D. M. (1985). *Action Science.* San Francisco: Jossey-Bass.

Balcazar, F., Keys, C., & Suarez-Balcazar, Y. (2001). Empowering Latinos with disabilities to address issues of independent living and disability rights: A capacity-building approach. *Journal of Prevention and Intervention in the Community, 21,* 53-70.

Balcazar, F., Keys, C., Kaplan, D., & Suarez-Balcazar, Y. (1998). Participatory action research and people with disabilities: Principles and challenges. *Canadian Journal of Rehabilitation, 12,* 105-112.

Beer, D., & Helfrich, C. (1996). Chicago Homeless Head Start Demonstration Project Evaluation, University of Illinois at Chicago, Department of Occupational Therapy.

Blake, H., & Moore, E. (2000). Partners share the credit for the partnerships accomplishments. In K. Connors & S.D. Seifer (Eds.), *Partnership perspectives, 1* (2), (pp. 65-70). San Francisco, CA: Community-Campus Partnerships for Health.

Braveman, B., Helfrich, C., & Fisher, G. S. (2001). Developing and maintaining community partnerships within a 'scholarship of practice.' *Education for Occupational Therapy in Health Care, 15 (1/2),* 109-125.

Carr, K. (2002). Building bridges and crossing borders: Using service learning to overcome cultural barriers to collaboration between science and education departments. *School Science and Mathematics, 102 (6),* 285-298.

Charlton, J. (1998). *Nothing about us without us: Disability oppression and empowerment.* Berkeley, CA: University of California Press.

Connors, K., & Seifer, S. D. (2000). *Partnership perspectives, 1* (2). San Francisco, CA: Community-Campus Partnerships for Health.

Cross, T., Bazron, B., Dennis, K., & Isaacs, M. (1989). Towards a culturally competent system of care. Washington, DC. George Town University Child Development Center, CASSP Technical Assistance Center.

Freire, P. (1970). Pedagogy of the Oppressed. New York: Herder and Herder.

Foster-Fishman, P., Berkowitz, S., Lounsbury, D., Jacobson, S., & Allen, N. (2001). Building collaborative capacity in community coalitions: A review and integrative framework. *American Journal of Community Psychology, 29*, 241-261.

Gills, D. C., Butler, M., Rose, A., & Bivens, S. (2001). Collaborative research and action in communities: Partnership building in the Chicago empowerment zone. In M. Sullivan & J. G. Kelly (Eds.), *Collaborative Research: University and Community Partnership* (pp. 25-44). Washington, DC: APHA.

Greenberg, J. S., Howard, D., & Desmond, S. (2003). A community-campus partnership for health: The Seat Pleasant-University of Maryland Health Partnership. *Health Promotion Practice, 4*, 393-401.

Hammel, J., Finlayson, M., Kielhofner, G., Helfrich, C., & Peterson, E. (2002). Educating Scholars of Practice: An Approach to Preparing Tomorrow's Researchers. *Occupational Therapy in Health Care, 15* (1/2), 157-176.

Harper, G. W., Lardon, C., Rappaport, J., Bangi, A., Contreras, R., & Pedraza, A. (2004). Community narratives: The use of narrative ethnography in participatory community research. In L. A. Jason, C. Keys, Y. Suarez-Balcazar, R. Taylor, M. Davis, J. Durlak, & D. Isenberg. (Eds.), *Participatory Community Research: Theories and Methods in Action* (199-217). Washington, DC. American Psychological Association.

Harper, G. W., & Salina, D. (2000). Building collaborative partnerships to improve community-based HIV prevention research: The university-CBO collaborative (UCCP) model. *Journal of Prevention & Intervention in the Community, 19*, 1-20.

Helfrich, C. (1997). *Homeless mothers' experience of transitional housing: An ethnographic study.* Unpublished Dissertation. PhD Public Health Sciences-Community Health, The University of Illinois at Chicago, Chicago.

Jackson, R. S., & Reddick, B. (1999). The African American church and university partnerships: Establishing lasting collaborations. *Health Education and Behavior, 26, 663-674.*

Jason, L. A., Keys, C. B., Suarez-Balcazar, Y., Taylor, R. R., & Davis, M. I. (2004). *Participatory Community Research: Theories and Methods in Action.* Washington, D. C.: American Psychological Association.

Lewin, K. (1946). Action research and minority problems. *Journal of Social Issues, 2,* 34-46.

Linton, S. (1998). Disability Studies/Not Disability Studies. In S. Linton, *Claiming Disability: Knowledge and Identity* (pp. 132-156). NY: New York University Press.

Longmore, P. K. (1995). "The Second Phase: From Disability Rights to Disability Culture." *Disability Rag & Resource, Sept./Oct.* Retrieved March 15, 2004, from http://www.independentliving.org/docs3/longm95.html

Longmore, P., & Umanksy, L. (2001). *The New Disability History.* New York: New York University Press.

Longmore, P. (2003). *Why I burned my book and other essays on disability.* Philadelphia, PA: Temple University Press.

Mattessich, P., & Monsey, B. (1992). *Collaboration: What makes it work.* St. Paul, MN: Amherst Wilder Foundation.

Nelson, G., Prillettensky, I., & MacGillivary, H. (2001). Building value-based partnerships: Toward solidarity with oppressed groups. *American Journal of Community Psychology, 29,* 649-677.

Oliver, M. (1996). The social model in context. *Understanding Disability from Theory to Practice* (pp. 30-42). New York: St. Martin's Press.

Panet-Raymond, J. (1992). Partnership: Myth or reality? *Community Development Journal, 27,* 156-65.

Perkins, D. D., & Wandersman, A. (1990). "You'll have to work to overcome our suspicions": The benefits and pitfalls of research with community organizations. *Social Policy, 20,* 32-41.

Prilleltensky, I. (2001). Value-based praxis in community psychology: Moving toward social justice and social action. *American Journal of Community Psychology, 29,* 747-778.

Riger, S. (2001). Working together: Challenges in collaborative research. In M. Sullivan & J. G. Kelly (Eds.), *Collaborative Research: University and Community Partnership* (pp. 25-44). Washington, DC: APHA.

Sanstad, K. H., Stall, R., Goldstein, E., Everett, W., & Brousseau, R. (1999). Collaborative community research consortium: A model for HIV prevention. *Health Education and Behavior, 26* (2), 171-184.

Selener, D. (1997). *Participatory action research and social change.* Ithaca: The Cornell Participatory Action Research Network.

Stewart, E. (2000). Thinking through others. In J. Rappaport & E. Seidman (Eds.), *Handbook of Community Psychology* (pp. 725-736). New York: Kluwer Academic.

Suarez-Balcazar, Y., Davis, M. I., Ferrari, J., Nyden, P., Olson, B., Alvarez, J., Molloy, P., & Toro, P. (2004). University-Community partnerships: A framework and an exemplar. In L. A. Jason, C. B. Keys, Y. Suarez-Balcazar, R. R. Taylor, & M. I. Davis, *Participatory Community Research* (pp. 105-120). Washington, D.C.: the American Psychological Association.

Suarez-Balcazar, Y., Durlak, J. A., & Smith, C. (1994). Multicultural training practices in community psychology programs. *American Journal of Community Psychology, 22,* 785-798.

Suarez-Balcazar, Y., Harper, G., & Lewis R. (2005). An interactive and contextual model of Community-University partnerships. *Health Education & Behavior.*

Suarez-Balcazar, Y., Muñoz, J., & Fisher G. (in press). Culturally competent university-community partnerships for Occupational Therapy Scholarship and Practice. In G. Kielhofner (Ed.). *Scholarship in Occupational Therapy: Methods of Inquiry for Enhancing Practice.* Philadelphia: F. A. Davis Company.

Suarez-Balcazar, Y., & Orellana-Damacela, L. (1999). A university-community partnership for empowerment evaluation in a community housing organization. *Sociological Practice: A Journal of Clinical and Applied Sociology, 1,* 115-132.

Suarez-Balcazar, Y., Orellana-Damacela, L., Portillo, N., Sharma, A., & Lanum, M. (2003). Implementing an outcomes model in the participatory evaluation of community initiatives. *Journal of Prevention and Intervention in the Community, 26* (2), 5-25.

Tandom, S. D., Azelton, S. L., & Kelly, J. G. (1998). Constructing a tree for community leaders: Contexts and process in collaborative inquiry. *American Journal of Community Psychology, 26,* 669-696.

Taylor, R. T., Hammel, J., & Braveman, B. (2004). Developing and evaluating community-based services through participatory action research: Two case examples. *American Journal of Occupational Therapy, 58 (1),* 73-82.

Thompson, L. S., Story, M., & Butler, G. (2003). Use of a university-community collaboration model to frame issues and set an agenda for strengthening a community. *Health Promotion Practice,* 4 (4), 385-392.

Velde, B. P., & Wittman, P. P. (2001). Helping occupational therapy students and faculty develop cultural competence. *Occupational Therapy in Health Care, 13,* 23-32

Walens, D., Helfrich, C. A., Aviles, A., & Horita, L. (2001). Assessing needs and developing interventions with new populations: A community process of collaboration. *Occupational Therapy in Mental Health,* 16 (3/4), 71-95.

Young, I. M. (1990). *Justice and the politics of difference.* Princeton. NJ: Princeton University Press.

The Practice-Scholar Program:
An Academic-Practice Partnership
to Promote the Scholarship
of "Best Practices"

Patricia Crist, PhD, OTR/L, FAOTA
Jaime Phillip Muñoz, PhD, OTR/L, FAOTA
Anne Marie Witchger Hansen, MS, OTR/L
Jeryl Benson, MS, OTR/L, BCP
Ingrid Provident, EdD, OTR/L

SUMMARY. Faculty-practitioner partnerships that address mutually established, practice-relevant priorities have great potential to bridge academy and practice. Each partner has a different purpose or mission but together embracing mutually beneficial opportunities through sustainable partnerships, exponentially increases the outcomes that could result.

The purpose of this paper is to report the evolution of a new program, called the Practice-Scholar Program at Duquesne University. The goal was to develop new partnerships between practice and our Department

Patricia Crist is Chair and Professor, Jaime Phillip Muñoz is Associate Professor, Anne Marie Witchger Hansen is Instructor and Practice-Scholar Program Coordinator, Jeryl Benson is Instructor, and Ingrid Provident is Assistant Professor and Fieldwork Coordinator, all with Duquesne University, Department of Occupational Therapy, 600 Forbes Avenue, Pittsburgh, PA 15282-0020.

[Haworth co-indexing entry note]: "The Practice-Scholar Program: An Academic-Practice Partnership to Promote the Scholarship of 'Best Practices'." Crist, Patricia et al. Co-published simultaneously in *Occupational Therapy in Health Care* (The Haworth Press, Inc.) Vol. 19, No. 1/2, 2005, pp. 71-93; and: *The Scholarship of Practice: Academic-Practice Collaborations for Promoting Occupational Therapy* (ed: Patricia Crist, and Gary Kielhofner) The Haworth Press, Inc., 2005, pp. 71-93. Single or multiple copies of this article are available for a fee from The Haworth Document Delivery Service [1-800-HAWORTH, 9:00 a.m. - 5:00 p.m. (EST). E-mail address: docdelivery@haworthpress.com].

Available online at http://www.haworthpress.com/web/OTHC
doi:10.1300/J003v19n01_06

to support mutual interests in teaching, research and service focusing on the scholarship of occupational therapy 'best practices' in a variety of settings. These 'best practice' sites are to develop model programs in occupational therapy stressing occupation-based practice, application of evidence in clinical decision-making and embed scholarship activities into their every day practice. The selection, development and sustenance of our Practice-Scholar program and our first four partnership sites are described in this paper. Our Practice-Scholars sites have been at a collaborative speech-language/occupational therapy pediatric clinic, and at three community sites: three day-care sites in a marginalized underserved community; a homeless shelter for women; and the county jail.

This paper describes how faculty have woven the Practice-Scholar program into our teaching, research and service responsibilities while helping our Practice-Scholars develop 'best practices.' Faculty, practitioner, and students benefits are described. Both the funding and outcomes from the Practice-Scholar program will be presented. Finally, new developments, modifications and challenges in sustaining these Practice-Scholar partnerships and scholarship of practice activities are discussed. *[Article copies available for a fee from The Haworth Document Delivery Service: 1-800-HAWORTH. E-mail address: <docdelivery@haworthpress. com> Website: <http://www.HaworthPress.com> © 2005 by The Haworth Press, Inc. All rights reserved.]*

KEYWORDS. Faculty, partnerships, scholarship, evidence-based practice

In 1999-2000, the Department of Occupational Therapy faculty at Duquesne University in Pittsburgh, Pennsylvania, recognized that an innovative opportunity existed to partner with occupational therapy practice to promote the profession in the areas of "best practices." A 'best practice' in occupational therapy would be occupation- and evidence-based and the practitioners would be engaged in research related to their practice as well as fieldwork education to prepare future practitioners with similar skill sets. Practitioners in these settings would be motivated, like the faculty, to promote the profession through modeling 'best practice' approaches in their practice settings including engaging in a scholarly approach to practice. Best practice partnerships that reflected the mutual needs of both the academic campus and practice could enhance both partners' responsibilities and activities.

These relationships evolve over time and emerge out of shared vision, agreed upon mission, values, goals and measurable outcomes (Waddock & Walsh, 1999; Cauley, 2000; Braveman, Helfrich, & Fisher, 2001). Effective partnerships are characterized by mutual trust and respect, genuineness and commitment to a common goal (Waddock & Walsh, 1999). Often these partnerships begin with conversations between faculty and community leaders, sharing interests, needs and resources. As the process continues, a formal collaboration begins to take shape based on a particular need. A common focus and vision is developed as each partner searches to identify their role, purpose, balance of power and resources (Connolly, 1999).

Duquesne University faculty realized the learning potential and relevance of developing these partnerships and using the natural environment as a resource for addressing relevant practice concerns and providing a new direction in student education. Faculty desired student learning in everyday contexts where students could learn from natural not contrived or modeled learning activities such as happened frequently in the classroom laboratories. Traditionally, faculty engage the community to identify subjects to participate in studies that were important to the faculty researcher but had little relevance to the daily life concerns of community members. Once the research or service program being evaluated was over, the professorate withdrew back to the "ivory tower" to publish, leaving the community feeling abused as a result of service withdrawal. Waddock and Walsh (1999) state that the community, the university and the students benefit when faculty emerge from the "ivory tower" and establish community partnerships. They suggest this partnership will change their typical practice of instruction and scholarship. Suggestions for change may include altering the way courses are designed and delivered, altering how the learner sees their future role within the community and changing the way faculty think about scholarship.

By answering practice questions relevant to everyday occupational therapy contexts, meaningful contemporary health issues can be addressed and provide evidence to support the practice of occupational therapy. Since many faculty are given time to do scholarship as integral to their role and our profession certainly needed evidence to support our practice contentions, our faculty saw a valuable, multi-faceted opportunity in promoting the scholarship of practice.

While our curriculum had a strong occupation-based practice focus, students seldom saw the use of occupation-based practice during fieldwork. Faculty felt that 'best practices' in education resulted in continuity across all learning, from classroom to clinic, and that students had the right to experience congruity between instruction and practice. Plus, until they saw occupation-based practice during fieldwork, the likelihood of students offering occupational-based practice as an entry-level practitioner was poor. More specifically, Waddock and Walsh (1999) suggested that altering the way courses are designed and delivered changes how the learner sees their future role within the community. Students trained within 'best practice' settings would have a set of skills to provide leadership in addressing critical issues in health care.

Our students clearly value 'learning with meaning' or in other words, developing professional skills and abilities that make a meaningful contribution to practice. Our students report enhanced motivation, skill development and satisfaction from learning in actual practice environments. For instance, practicing a screening tool at a day-care center that used the information to monitor children's development was favored over bringing children into a lab for assessment practice. Developing a grant for a community agency to create an occupational therapy program was preferred over writing a business plan for a fictitious department in administration class. Doing a walk through a marginalized community and interviewing key community leaders to identify potential ways OT could serve a community was more instructive than watching a video on diversity. Finally, while students learned basic research competencies on campus, they seldom observed practitioners engaged in studies of practice. This led students to believe that practitioners did not embrace the role of clinical researcher, and that research is an activity that only faculty, not practitioners, do. Further, while they recognized that the future of their profession rested on creating practice-relevant evidence, beyond lecture experiences, they did not understand how scholarship could be embedded in everyday practice to address this concern.

Faculty-practitioner partnerships based on collaborative problem-solving, shared student preparation, and interest in applied research activities that address mutually established, practice-relevant priorities have great potential to bridge academy and practice. This approach had potential to re-frame a previous way of engagement into a 'win-win' partnership for both parties with the benefits extended to students and our profession. Each partner had a different purpose or mission but together embracing mutually beneficial opportunities through sustainable partnerships, exponentially increased the outcomes that could result.

The purpose of this paper is to report the evolution of a new program, called the Practice-Scholar Program at Duquesne University. The goal was to develop new partnerships between practice and our Department to support mutual interests in teaching, research and service focusing on the scholarship of occupational therapy 'best practices' in a variety of settings. The role, 'practice-scholar,' was coined by our faculty to mirror the role, 'teacher-scholar,' used on our campus to reflect faculty performance expectations. Faculty at Duquesne are focused equally on both "teaching and the conduct of research and other scholarly activities related to the development of new knowledge within their discipline" (*Duquesne University Faculty Handbook*, 2005, p. 26). However, faculty were committed to helping practitioners achieve this Practice-Scholar goal, too, including providing professional development consultations and collaborative activities.

The selection, development and maintenance of our Practice-Scholar sites through partnerships will be delineated in this paper. A section will be devoted to show how faculty have woven the Practice-Scholar program into our teaching, research and service responsibilities. Finally new developments, modifications and challenges in sustaining this model will be discussed.

BACKGROUND

The external context for the development of the Practice-Scholar program had many supportive structures unfolding such as Boyer's *Scholarship Reconsidered* (1990), Donald Schön's *Reflective Practitioner,* and Campus Compact's focus on civic engagement and service-learning through campus-community partnerships to balance the missions of workforce development, college preparation and education for citizenship (Ravitch & Viteritti, 2001). Congruence with our University's purpose for faculty has already been discussed but also, our mission that states, " Duquesne serves God by serving students–through service to . . . the community." The faculty are commissioned to prepare leaders with professional expertise who are 'guided by consciences sensitive to the needs of society' (Duquesne University's Mission Statement, 2004).

Boyer's (1990) influential report through the Carnegie Foundation has resulted in many campus discussions to broaden the understanding of scholarship in order to better align faculty priorities and the missions of our colleges and universities and the knowledge development needed by our society at large. This re-alignment of academic expectations has resulted in more equal footing between funded and unfunded research, quantitative and qualitative approaches, efficacy and effectiveness studies, and basic and applied research, to name a few. Meaningfulness and value became as important to knowledge discovery as prestige and scientific control. Boyer's model resulted in a wider number of options for faculty to select research agenda and academic campuses that matched their values and desire to contribute to knowledge development in their field.

Donald Schön advocated that theory and practice were not hierarchically organized. However, each college or university chose the type of knowledge development desired and set about building institutional structures to declare these values in terms of policies, practices, supports and most importantly, faculty performance rewards. A major group of occupational therapy scholars and practitioners followed Donald Schön's work regarding reflective practice in the 80's and developed our understanding of clinical reasoning in occupational therapy practice (Fleming, 1991).

Campus Compact is a national organization focused on promoting the civic engagement of faculty and students through the scholarship of engagement. To broaden the conception of scholarship to include, the 'scholarship of engagement,' Rice (2003) proposed engaged pedagogy, community-based research and collaborative practice to correspond with the customary faculty responsibilities of teaching, research and service. Engaged pedagogy is service learning and learning communities focused on experiential, contextual, social and reflective learning. Community-based research reflects a local time and setting and utilizes community peers in a collaborative, multidirectional study. Collaborative practice is campus service to address concrete, protracted community-based problems to sustain healthy communities and quality of life. The scholarship of engagement requires faculty and campuses to support, legitimize and reward the scholarship of engagement if success is desired.

Now, occupational therapy faculty can find campuses that will value and reward a variety of scholarly work. Some campuses have a large array of options, others are more limited. Regardless, faculty are encouraged to learn their college's or university's values regarding the varying types of research. Faculty members should seek work on campuses that value and reward their preferred scholarship agenda. Similarly, an occupational therapy academic program housed at a college or university can create a valuable 'scholarship of practice' program unique to their setting and expectations.

For instance, the Occupational Therapy Department and the University of Illinois at Chicago has reported their 'Scholarship of Practice' program (Braveman, Helfich, & Fisher, 2001). In reviewing this publication, many of the guidelines for development and maintenance of successful partnerships with community organizations are useful and relevant. A formal presentation of their model at a day-long institute in Chicago in 2002 stimulated interest among occupational therapy program directors in establishing academic-community partnerships to support the scholarship of practice and to prepare practitioners for community-based practice. However, the majority of attendees felt that emulating this model was impossible because:

- their campuses did not have the flexibility of financial resources for new program development like this Research I University
- their setting did not have the requisite faculty capital
- their faculty did not possess the degrees to prepare them for major grant competition to fund a UIC approach to the scholarship of practice
- they did not have access to funded graduate students to provide support grant writing, literature searching, and service delivery
- the sustainability of the community programs was not possible for on-going relationships even though the UIC presenters stated that sites had secured their own funding.

Regardless, a majority of occupational therapy program directors felt that the scholarship of practice would be very motivating for their faculty and reflect their civic-mindedness but felt unable to translate the model into their setting. At the time of the UIC presentation, our Department was already well into its second year of the Practice-Scholar program which offered a different way to engage in the scholarship of practice Discussion between the UIC and Duquesne University after this presentation, indicated that a variety of scholarship of practice models would be valuable to maximize the match between occupational therapy educators and practitioners interests and resources.

VISIONING A NEW RESOURCE TO BENEFIT THE UNIVERSITY AND THE COMMUNITY

Our department envisions practice-scholar activities as possible within any setting where occupational therapy practice is occurring. In fact, a variety of 'best practice' sites is desired. Our goal is to be 'capacity-builders' for our students, partners in practice, practice-scholars and faculty through creating and engaging in the scholarship of 'best practices' in occupational therapy.

At the beginning of this specific initiative, three faculty with experience in community-based practice and motivation to establish community-based partnerships came together to pursue the practice-scholar program. Another practice-scholar program was initiated by a faculty member for children in our University's speech-language clinic.

As a core group of faculty experienced in community-based practice, three of us found ourselves in a professional community that for the most part had abandoned community service to provide medically-focused interventions in our huge medical and health sciences complex in Pittsburgh, Pennsylvania. About this same time, the profession started talking about occupational therapy entering new 'emerging areas of practice.' A meeting of our curriculum advisory committee consisted of area practice leaders. At this meeting, the practitioners urged the faculty to send students into the community to open community-based practice but warned us that we would not find revenue to sustain occupational therapy practices as there were very few reimbursement streams to support community-based practice.

The Duquesne faculty accepted the challenge presented by the curriculum advisory committee, which was enormous due to the lack of OTs already engaged in community-based practice locally, the way practice relied on the medical model to shape practice, and the funding challenge so that these activities could produce employment of practitioners. Our Practice-Scholar program was initiated in 2000 with the vision to demonstrate 'best practices' in occupational therapy through mutual partnerships that promoted practice, education, research and service. Our first practice-scholar sites were in pediatric out-patient and community-based occupational therapy.

DESCRIPTION OF INITIAL PRACTICE
SCHOLAR PROGRAMS

Though out-of-sequence, future text will be easier to deliver if the reader has knowledge of the partnerships that have evolved so far. This is an overview of each as extensive description is beyond this space. Current and future publications will be more explicit.

- *Good Beginnings:* The Good Beginnings Program is an integrated occupational therapy and speech-language pathology program staffed by one faculty from the Occupational Therapy and Speech-Language Pathology departments. The purpose of this program is to provide collaborative experiences for the students, provide direct integrated services to children and to provide clinical research opportunities for the faculty and the students (Benson, Williams, &

Stern, 2002). The clinic currently accepts students for level I field-work placements and/or independent study.

- *Quality Day Care:* The department secured its first grant through a partnership with the YMCA of Pittsburgh. This eighteen month federal grant supported the hiring of two Practice Scholars to provide sensory, social, and behavioral occupational therapy inventions to at-risk 0-5 year-olds. The Practice Scholars also recommended environmental adaptations and provided training for day care staff and developmental interventions for family support at three urban Y-Care Day Care sites.
- *Project Employ:* Bethlehem Haven, a shelter for women who are homeless, had created a one-stop shop to move women from homelessness back to community engagement and productivity. The worthy goal of this agency is to "eradicate homeless so that Bethlehem Haven can be closed" (personal communication with Executive Director, Marilyn Sullivan). The shelter had developed employment services for their residents through the Project Employ program as an essential element in their rehabilitation plan. However, before the development of this community-university partnership, Project Employ was not successful at providing pre-employment skill development or appropriate job placements for their clients. Now, Practice-Scholars at this site prepare and place formerly homeless woman and recently, men as well, in paid employment and provide life skills training to prevent a return to homelessness. The program is grant-funded by Allegheny County, HUD and private foundations and is in its fourth year.
- *Allegheny County Jail Community Re-Integration Project:* We offered to partner with Goodwill Industries of Pittsburgh to develop a comprehensive community re-integration and employment program for inmates who were within 6 months of leaving the county jail. The goal was to get these individuals employed and back into healthier living environments in order to prevent re-incarceration. Follow-up was 12 months post-release. Occupational therapy developed the living skills program and provided adaptation of individual employment situations to match specific needs of the program participants. A multidisciplinary team including leadership by two Practice-Scholars and, for one year, three occupational therapists, has successfully reduced recidivism with the major reason cited for these results, the work of occupational therapy (Crist, Fairman, Muñoz, Hansen, Sciulli, & Eggers, 2005). This program is in its fourth year.

The last three partnerships were all competitively grant funded on the first submission through the county and state. The funding agencies noted the value of the diversity of competencies and resources brought by the partnership, especially the presence of University-based occupational therapy as a significant asset in their award decisions.

IDENTIFYING SUITABLE PARTNERS

The faculty was not tied to any one method to identify potential partners, and was also open to others seeking us out. In fact, at least three different methods are already present. Initially, faculty strategically identified key agencies and talked with leadership in search of identifying mutual interests and desire to participate in our Practice-Scholar initiative. In recognition of the continuity we needed for Practice-Scholar program development, a faculty member was hired as the coordinator. This individual was given few other faculty responsibilities for one year except to stimulate the Practice-Scholar program with the primary activity to identify and nurture potential partners. Her success was so great that far sooner than expected we had to set priorities in our partnership pursuits, as once discovered, the community was hungry for occupational therapy services. One frustration was the number of agencies who wanted OT after our contact but who could not find funding for practice-scholar activities immediately. Likewise, faculty quickly became aware of the intensity of support needed to support the professional development of practices scholars and their programs transitioning to 'best practice' settings. This did open doors to creative collaborations with students through classes, fieldwork and volunteer activities to be discussed later.

Initially, a very productive meeting was held with the Allegheny County director of the Department of Health and Human Services (DHHS) that ended in the realization of the congruence between their agency's strategic objectives and our occupational therapy goals. The department leadership facilitated numerous meetings for our faculty and key individuals inside their department as well as with external agencies who they felt could support our Practice-Scholar agenda. This service was important as we learned that DHHS did not coordinate any of the services they offered; they were a broker for funding ones offered by others, primarily non-profit organizations, that met their mission and purposes. Early on, they even invited us to write a request for proposals for a major Work Incentive Act (WIA) funding program they were planning to release because it aligned so closely with occupational therapy philosophy. However, we refused this offer as we wanted to be a competitor for these funds! In fact, this funding soon supported the goals for our Bethlehem Haven and Goodwill partnerships.

For Good Beginnings, the faculty member desired to practice as part of her faculty role and developed this service through a relationship with a faculty member in our Department of Speech, Language, and Pathology. The conceptual model was to provide collaborative services, occupational therapy and speech-language pathology services jointly, for children. Since the faculty is already salaried, no additional funding is needed for this site. We were able to work within the existing infrastructure of the Speech, Language, and Hearing Clinic, using equipment and resources that were already available within both departments and using clinic space in the SLP department (Benson, Williams, & Stern, 2002). Speech has agreed to let us use their billing system to collect fees for no cost until our volume significantly impacts their current fee management processes. During the second year of the program a small grant was secured to support the development of the program. The grant and revenue monies have been used to support Good Beginnings and faculty development.

While being the YMCA Director of our University's public day care center, the current director of all YMCA day care programs increased her awareness of occupational therapy's expertise in person-environment issues when OT students came to her daycare to screen children as a way to practice assessment skills. When she became aware of new state funding to support changes in her daycare centers, she approached us and asked to partner with us on the grant. The YMCA wrote and submitted the grant and were a subcontractor overseeing and supporting our two Practice-Scholars. The Y project was funded for 2 years and no new funds were found to continue but much had been accomplished and learned.

Communities are aware of their needs and seek universities as one of the valuable resources for addressing their concerns. Communities value partnerships with academic programs when programs or research addresses issues or provides solutions relevant to their population and are sustainable after the project ends (Checkoway, 2001).

In the community, capacity-building was initiated with community partners to provide the equal opportunity to identify pressing problems in their terms regarding their community's unique quality of life challenges. Our community partners lead the problem identification process and then together, we collaboratively design, implement and now, maintain occupational therapy services that transform local communities. From these efforts, the Goodwill and Bethlehem Haven projects transformed into grant-funded partnerships. We sought out the Goodwill after reviewing three other potential partners as we realized we could not meet all the anticipated goals stated by the funding source. Goodwill, since they would provide the majority of service agreed to subcontract with us for occupational therapy. With Bethlehem Haven, we learned that the funding source preferred that we be the contractor for this service and we agreed to move forward after the Haven stated they wanted to move ahead with fully implementing this program.

Early in the uncovering of mutually identified needs and the development of these Practice Scholar partnerships, we discovered the potential for other university programs, faculty and students to contribute to these developing projects. Our community partners enthusiastically supported our invitation to participate in a "Community University Conversation." Twenty-five faculty members from thirteen academic programs met with ten community agency representatives from our two practice scholar sites to share an overview of their agency and/or academic program's assets and needs. Several other community-university partnerships evolved from this conversation including the development of a pastoral ministry internship at Bethlehem Haven and a music therapy internship at the Allegheny County jail.

CREATING A NEW INTERNAL STRUCTURE TO SUPPORT THE PROGRAM

At the beginning of the Practice-Scholar program, several agreements were made regarding the operation of this program within our University. We agreed to not use University operating funds to support this program unless related to classroom teaching or fieldwork. The dean of our school agreed that our practice-scholar sites did not have to be considered part of the School's practice plan which meant that we did not have to generate revenue or share acquired management fees or indirect dollars with the practice plan. Second, he agreed to name practice-scholars as non-tenure track, clinical faculty appointments affording them the privileges and benefits of academic faculty immediately. Finally, all practice-scholar activities were to be self-supporting minimizing the drain on our current operational budget. We did not want our operational budget cut-back because of this alternative funding stream. If indirect funding was available through the grants, we were to request the maximum allowable in our budgets and all indirect monies were subject to the published revenue share allocation between the University, School and principal investigator. If an administrative or other management fee was provided, then the revenue from this source would go directly to the department to support scholarly and/or grant-related activities. To date, not one of our grants has exceeded 8% indirect or administrative fee allowance on the bottom line. Finally, our administration, Office of Sponsored Research, Risk Management and Dean's Office created new financial and administrative systems to beneficially support our program.

FUNDING THE PRACTICE-SCHOLAR INITIATIVE

To be selected as a community partner, at minimum, the partner had to support the teaching and scholarship goals of the Practice-Scholar Program and agree to support the development of a 'best practices' occupational therapy program. Our partners and our community connections helped us identify potential external funding to support the Practice-Scholar program. Table 1 identifies funding sources for our Practice-Scholar sites so far.

With all funding, we negotiated our fair share of indirect or administration fees on our portion of the budget, be it a subcontract or contract. This is not a standard and must be negotiated as soon as possible, preferable before budget development.

For up to the first 3 years of funding, Practice-Scholars were faculty employed through the University. This was valuable as the management fees came to the department to support various activities in return for

TABLE 1. Practice-Scholar Program Grants

Title	Funding Source	Total
Goodwill Industries "Best Practice Demonstration Projects/Clinical Scholar Program" (3 years)	City of Pittsburgh and Allegheny County	$457,657.00
"Community Re-Integration Project" (1 year)	City of Pittsburgh and Allegheny County	$91,497.00
Bethlehem Haven "Project Employ Program" (1 year)	Housing and Urban Development	$55,753.00
Bethlehem Haven "Project Employ Program" (3 years)	Allegheny County Department of Human Services–Special Populations Grant	$129,170.00
Good Beginnings: Supplies for Best Practices (1 year)	RSHS Faculty Practice Plan (Internal)	$5,000.00
	Grand total:	$739,077.00

faculty time not reimbursed by these county grants. However, over time these funds became nearly non-existent do to funding cut-backs in this category or as the result of decisions by the partners to pay for staff instead of management fees when times were tight. At the end of the third year, the Department transferred our subcontract or contract back to the partner. While we are staying involved with the sites from a Practice-Scholar perspective, relinquishing the contract simplified management processes and reduced costs to the University that were no longer being covered. Although the Practice-Scholars preferred to be University employees, all other Practice-Scholar activities seemed accomplishable without contractual arrangements. Thus, in the current and fourth year of two projects, a faculty member vested in each specific site has become the primary contact to ensure continuing engagement with our Practice-Scholar sites for the purposes that originated the program. External funding when beneficial to the department is good but this was never a requirement of the practice-scholar partnerships.

The faculty creating the Practice-Scholar program became aware of the two typical reactions by community leaders regarding occupational therapy as we sought partners. First, partners were surprised to learn about our array of professional competencies as many thought that the only individuals we worked with were persons with strokes and hand injuries. With a broadened view of our practice, community agencies saw the alignment with occupational therapy clearer. The second largest response received from community contacts was not favorable. In the 90's, those who tried to hire occupational therapists found applicants arrogant, self-serving and willingly offering competitive salary demands typical in other market sectors. Most community leaders were appalled and sought other professionals who were more compassionate and reasonable. Many still desired occupational therapy and, as a result gave us an opportunity to share our interests. As a result of these two factors, we incorporated educational opportunities regarding the breadth of OT service, with specific reference to their interests, early in contacting potential partners. Many times we did searches of our professional literature prior to our first meeting to discover systematic concerns, shared interests, and working programs already in place.

DEVELOPING PRACTICE SCHOLARS

The evolution of our practice scholar program is a journey in collaboration that has required both the faculty and the practitioners to stretch and challenge themselves in new roles and ways of working. Regular meetings were a key to establishing the relationships. Initial meetings focused on finding common ground and on defining best practice at each community site. Our goals for best practice programming at each community scholar site included:

- to establish programming that was evidenced based and outcomes oriented
- to maximize interdisciplinary collaboration
- to establish local, state, and national reputation for practice scholarship
- to generate scholarship that contributes to occupational therapy body of knowledge

Our practice scholars voiced concerns that they needed to increase their knowledge of outcomes research methods and to develop strategies for integrating habits of scholarship into daily routines and treatment contexts that emphasized and valued the delivery of service over scholarship. Regular meeting times were established that provided a structured time to address the practice scholars' requests for increased knowledge and skills and as a way to begin to develop the habits of scholarship. These meetings solidified our relationships. Practitioners educated the faculty about the day-to-day realities of their programs, the outcome expectations of their primary funders and the intricacies of interdisciplinary work when the familiarity of working with physical, speech and other rehabilitation therapists was replaced by working with probation and parole officers, jail guards, and community activists. Over the next several months the habits of scholarship were supported by:

- examining literature together
- keeping a running log of potential research questions
- problem-solving programmatic issues
- reviewing qualitative and quantitative research designs
- defining how directed research studies would compliment but differ from the data their funding agencies required
- having the practice scholars recognize and articulate researchable questions

The practice scholars signaled their readiness to move to the next stage of application when they began initiating proposals for scholarly projects. Collectively, the group prioritized preliminary research questions, wrote research proposals and completed the Duquesne University IRB process. Faculty efforts shifted to supporting the efforts of collecting literature to support the development of these proposals, suggesting and critiquing research design proposals and providing crash courses in outcomes measurement and IRB procedures. The efforts were time consuming and faculty would frequently joke that the practice scholars were well on their way to a clinical doctorate degree.

Another major focus of the collaboration at this time was to support the dissemination of these emerging practice programs through the presentation of scholarly posters and papers at state and national conference. Faculty partnered with the practice scholars to submit proposals and ultimately deliver scholarly presentation at state and national conferences. Additionally, the practice scholars were mentored to publish. These efforts began with feature pieces in *OT Practice*, evolved to a program description in the *Mental Health Special Interest Quarterly* (Eggers, Scuilli, Gaguzis, & Muñoz, 2003) and grew to manuscript publications and submissions to peer-reviewed journals (Eggers, Sciulli, Gaguzis, & Muñoz, 2003; Benson, Williams, & Stern, 2002; Eggers, Muñoz, Sciulli, & Crist, in press; Muñoz, Reichenbach & Hansen, in press). The journey continues. Some research projects are underway and others are in various stages of design. The relationship between the university faculty and the practice scholars has developed to a point where a more comprehensive research agenda that integrates the practice-scholars, individual faculty, and student scholarship can be pursued.

PRACTICE-SCHOLAR OUTCOMES

As already described, our goal for this program was to nurture the development of occupational therapists delivering 'best practice' sites that provided instructional resources for students, scholarship access for faculty and provided at minimum, the professional development of a new generation of practitioners. Earlier, funding success was described. In Table 2, major Practice-Scholar outcomes are listed.

Some of these activities are self-explanatory, such as practice-scholars offering specialty lectures and labs including bringing some of their clients in for panels. This table indicates the number of our Practice-Scholar sites that participated in this activity (P-S), the number of students who benefited and if the activity occurred across more than one semester. The extensiveness of the activity is not represented but typically, if a semester is represented, it means that there was weekly contact with P-S site for no less than 6 weeks but as much as the entire semester.

TABLE 2. Practice-Scholar Program Outcomes: The First 4 Years

Teaching:

Practice-Scholar contributions

- P-S serve as problem-based learning instructor (1 P-S; 10 students)
- P-S grade student-generated assessment documentation gathered at their site (1P-S; 22 students)
- P-S assist faculty in administering and scoring a pediatric practical examination (1P-S; 22 students)
- Guest lecture on psychosocial aspects of spinal cord injury (pre-PS OT work role) (1P-S; 29 students)
- Guest lecture on community practice (3 P-S; 57 students; 2 semesters)
- Panel discussion in administration course regarding program development strategies (2 P-S; 29 students)
- Panel discussion on competencies for community practice (2P-S; 53 students; four semesters)
- Guest lecture on finding and maintaining funding (1 P-S; 29 students; two semesters)
- Guest lecture on dealing with difficult patients/clients (2 P-S; 13 students)
- Presented seminar on community-based research projects (2 P-S; 25 students; two semesters)
- P-S served as informants for 4 qualitative student research projects (2 P-S; 18 students)

Student Learning

- Students practice interviewing skills with former jail inmates (1 P-S; 29 students)
- Students complete assessment/documentation exercises with children (1 P-S; 22 students)
- Students complete psychosocial assessment/documentation exercises (2 P-S; 34 students; 2 semesters)
- Students completed advanced topic course in psychosocial practice at P-S sites (1 P-S; 2 students)
- Student on fieldwork completed a site-related applied research proposal as part of another course (3 P-S; 5 fieldwork students)
- Independent study on OT theory and practice related to site population (P-S; 1 student)
- Students designed and implemented a new intervention group (P-S; 1 student)
- Numerous portfolio evidence regarding competencies in specific areas of service delivery that encourage self-reflection and benefit job searching

Fieldwork

- Level I fieldwork (3 P-S; 14 students)
- Level II fieldwork (3 P-S; 5 students)

Scholarly Activities :*

- 4 presentations at state conference
- 1 poster at state conference
- 1 panel at national conference
- 1 paper at national conference
- 1 poster at national conference
- 4 manuscripts, published or accepted in professional journals; 1 manuscript in review
- 2 articles in *OT Practice* describing our practice-scholar program
- Article in *Mental Health Special Interest Section Quarterly*

TABLE 2 (continued)

Service/Service Learning

- Students administer COPM, the tool administered to all inmates, as part of class (1P-S; 12 students)
- Students complete 2 semester-long, service learning projects at Practice-Scholar sites (3 P-S; 11 students; 4 semesters)
- Students complete pediatric lab group sessions 1x/week for several weeks. (1 P-S; 24 students)
- Students write draft grant proposal as part of course to expand programming (1 P-S; 3 students)
- 3 student volunteers in program (2 P-S)

Practice

- Contributed to development of first job fair held inside jail
- Students observed treatment groups for a class (P-S; 2 students)
- 9 OTRS and 1 COTA have worked within our Practice-Scholar sites

*All are co-authored by faculty and practice-scholars except one poster and one manuscript.

INSTRUCTIONAL INNOVATION

While our practice-scholars provided specialty lectures in classes, a two semester clinical reasoning and fieldwork course had gradually developed a community service component where students paired with a self-selected community site. Across two semesters, they moved from a needs assessment offering an intervention program. Course feedback demonstrated not only the value of the learning experience but also, many agencies became aware of the value of occupational therapy in their settings and sought out the Department for assistance. Once major instructional innovation was an outcome from a later course in which students planned an occupational therapy program relevant to an assigned community site who desired occupational therapy services. This activity for the site transformed into preparing a universal grant application for the site. These student activities uncovered many leads to explore future Practice-Scholar opportunities. All these activities as well as each step toward creating the Practice-Scholar community-based program began with education of the community. The core faculty creating the Practice-Scholar program were aware of the typical reactions by community leaders regarding occupational therapy. They were surprised to learn about our array of competencies, as many thought all we worked with were persons with strokes and hand injuries.

FIELDWORK DEVELOPMENT

The importance of preparing students for clinical practice within the Practice Scholar sites, through fieldwork was seen as an important goal of the program. Comprehensive fieldwork programs were established at all of the practice scholar sites. These fieldwork programs were created through meetings between the academic fieldwork coordinator and the practice scholars, whereby unique fieldwork opportunities were structured at each of the sites (Provident & Joyce-Gaguzis, 2005).

Several Duquesne University students were placed at these sites for either level I and/or level II fieldwork placements. To date, 5 Duquesne students have completed level II placements (2 at YMCA, 2 at the Jail and 1 at Bethlehem Haven). A greater number of students, 14 total, have completed Level I rotations (6 at Bethlehem Haven, 4 at the Jail, and 4 at Good Beginnings). It was originally hoped that a greater percentage of our students would be placed at these sites for fieldwork opportunities, however, students had expressed a desire to go to fieldwork sites that they were not familiar with, stating that they felt they understood and had been exposed to the practice scholar sites through a number of curricular experiences at these sites throughout the course of their didactic and laboratory experiences.

The Practice-Scholar sites are highly desired to train Level II fieldwork students because of the quality services provided. We are encouraging the practice scholars to contact other schools and pursue fieldwork contracts to meet this need. We have agreed to write a letter of support to accompany their inquiry information.

STUDENT ENGAGEMENT

As was seen in Table 2, students have benefited through this program in terms of learning community-based and specialty practice services from needs assessment to grant writing as well as interventions. Much has been in the form of service learning where their learning has contributed to a site-identified need. They have observed and even participated in, embedded research activities in practice and the value of academic-practice partnerships as a form of enhanced collegial relationships that can support professional development and promote occupational practice through innovative program development and evidence. Through classroom and modeling, students learn how to partner with practitioners, agencies and provide population-based services.

Most importantly, students have seen how a vision can be converted to reality in both emerging areas of practice but also, in a locale that essentially had medical and school-based occupational therapy services only. In many instances, they have had opportunities to see their faculty as teacher-scholars, practitioners and leaders beyond the classroom and in some instances, partnered to create system change. From our venture into marginalized communities, a significant change in the ethos and closed-mindedness of our students has occurred from one so fearful to walk into unfamiliar marginalized communities to one where they seek conversations with community representatives for joint problem-solving. Lastly, these activities have resulted in excellent evidence in their professional portfolios supporting real life problem-solving and skills development, not to mention continuous reflection on their professional development and acquired professional self-efficacy. During post-Level II fieldwork capstone coursework, students frequently showcase their learning from this specific program. Most telling is the number of practitioners who interview our students and contact faculty to not only state that their portfolios were extraordinarily helpful during the interview process but that students had real evidence of service delivery competencies well beyond those typically acquired through classroom and fieldwork activities. Our students, as entrepreneurs in areas where few OTs have ventured, are just beginning to emerge.

PROGRAMMATIC TRANSITIONS AND MODIFICATIONS ALONG THE WAY

With any innovative program, the experience is more a journey than a directed process. As new learning or challenges occur, so must adaptations. Much of our journey is chronicled above; however, a few tidbits remain to be told. First, we originally appointed the Practice-Scholars as clinical faculty but as time progressed, we realized that this did not accurately describe their activities and when University processes such as annual performance evaluation came forward, significant challenges were met, practice-scholar activities were too disparate with traditional faculty expectations. While practice-scholars desired to be named faculty, the administrative track was more accurate placement. With enhanced integration of practice-scholars into the teaching enterprise and/or role development as productive clinical scholars, appointment to the faculty track is possible. All are eligible for adjunct faculty appointment when activities relate uniquely and positively to teaching activities and scholarly productivity.

From the start, we sought to have certified occupational therapy assistants (COTAs) in our practice-scholar programs and to date, one was employed for a short duration to provide on-going regular services. Finding COTAs prepared and interested in this type of programming has been a challenge. Additionally, in our current sites where program development is intensive, funding is scarce, and the desire to be engaged scholars of practice is high, occupational therapists provide greater practice-scholar abilities.

NEW DEVELOPMENTS AND FUTURE GOALS

With the recent release from holding grant funds as ties to two of our current programs for reasons discussed already, a high desire is present to retain our academic-practice relationships. This new relationship is evolving as this is written. A faculty member has agreed to serve as the single-point of contact for each site. The faculty provides a conduit for coordination of teaching and research issues but also, has high interest in the program to address their own faculty responsibilities. Certainly, we recognize how much prior relationship-building supports a commitment by both to continue these mutually beneficial interactions.

To expand the types of practice-scholar sites and engage more of our master practitioners in the area, the faculty are discussing the implementation of a new seminar-approach to help current practitioners in more traditional settings, implement the practice-scholar model through a partnership with us that is congruent with our goals for this unique program.

CONCLUSION

In closing, we have chosen to cover the major steps and decisions in the development of our Practice-Scholar program. This program was and continues to be a journey with our current partners' base on flexibility, accountability and the pursuit of excellence. Events never took place in a linear fashion, and likely will never, as long as we adhere to the philosophy of practice partnerships.

As a result of the evolving Practice-Scholar program coupled with inventive faculty, the University views the department as innovators and leaders for current strategic initiatives in service learning, civic engagement, creative teaching excellence, meaningful community service, and academic leadership. In other terms, we are leading the scholarship of practice using a civic engagement philosophy aimed at creating graduates who have the skills to become practice-scholars, a new wave in practitioner competency.

ACKNOWLEDGMENT

The authors are indebted to the following individuals who are just a few of the many collaborators whose support has ensured the success of our Practice-Scholar Program from its inception: Bethlehem Haven: Practice-Scholars Diana Reichenbach, Sara ____, Andrea Patrick & Anna Lisa Wolfe along with Executive Director, Marilyn Sullivan; Goodwill Industries of Pittsburgh Practice Scholars John Scuilli, Mila Eggers McNutt, & Kelly Gazukis along with Eric Yenerall and Mike Oleck; YMCA of Pittsburgh: Lorelie Moser and Jackie Pillar along with Y ____ and finally, Diana Williams and Mikael Kimmelman, Chair, Department of Speech Language Pathology at Duquesne University. Each of these individuals left a handprint on our Practice-Scholar Program.

AUTHORS' NOTES

Unbeknownst to any of the following participants at the World Federation of Occupational Therapists meetings in Stockholm, two papers were presented using the term 'practice-scholar' on June, 27, 2002. Dr. Patricia Crist and Anne Marie Witchger Hansen presented a poster titled: "Practice-Scholar Program: Innovative Education Model Integrating Teaching, Scholarship & Practice" (poster) that created the initial draft for this manuscript. We had used this term since the inception of our program ande thought it was an original label for our practice-based, grant-supported staff. On the same day as our poster, Dr. Gary Kielhofner from the University of Illinois at Chicago used this term in his keynote address, titled, *Challenges and Directions for the Future of Occupational Therapy*, in which he recognized Kirsty Forsyth and Lynn Summerfield-Mann for first applying this term to clinicians and academics working together as part of the United Kingdom, Center for Outcomes Research and Education. While this appears to be an indicator of 'great minds thinking alike,' we want the readers to know that this is what happened and the term 'practice-scholar' was selected and used by these two separate, independently-evolving programs to uniquely describe individuals and/or associated activities in each.

REFERENCES

Benson, J. D., Williams, D. L., & Stern, P. (2002) The Good Beginnings Clinic: An Interdisciplinary Collaboration. *Occupational Therapy in Healthcare*, 16 (2/3): 21-37.

Boyer, E. L. (1990). *Scholarship reconsidered: Priorities of the Professorate*. New York: Carnegie Foundation for the Advancement of Teaching.

Braveman, B. H., Helfrich, C. A., & Fisher, G. S. (2001). Developing & maintaining community partnerships within a "scholarship of practice." *Occupational Therapy in Health Care*, 15 (1/2): 109-25.

Cauley, K. (2000). Partners have agreed-upon mission, values, goals and measurable outcomes for partnerships. *Partnership Perspectives*, I, 13-17.

Chockoway, B. (2001). Renewing the civic mission of the American Research University. *Journal of Higher Education*, 72 (2): 125-147.

Connolly, C. (2000). The partnership balances the power among partners and enables resources among partners to be share. *Partnership Perspectives*, I, 33-40.

Crist, P., Fairman, A., Muñoz, J. P., Hansen, AM. W., Sciulli, J., & Eggers, M. (2005). Education & Practice Collaboration: A Pilot Case Study Between A University Faculty and County Jail Practitioners. *Occupational Therapy in Health Care*, 19 (1/2): 193-210.

Duquesne University. (2005). *Duquesne University Faculty Handbook*. Pittsburgh, PA: Duquesne University.

Eggers, M., Muñoz, J. P., Sciulli, J. & Crist, P. A. (in press). The Community Reintegration Project: Occupational Therapy at Work in a County Jail. *Occupational Therapy in Health Care*.

Eggers, M., Sciulli, J., Gaguzis, K., & Muñoz, J. P. (2003, June). Enrichment Through occupation: The Allegheny County Jail project. *AOTA Mental Health Special Interest Section Quarterly*, 26, (2), 1-4.

Fleming, M. H. (1991) The therapist with a three track mind. *American Journal of Occupational Therapy*, 45, 1007-1014.

Muñoz, J. P., Reichenbach, D., & Witchger Hansen, A. (in press) Project Employ: Engineering hope and breaking down barriers to homelessness. *WORK-A Journal of Prevention, Assessment and Rehabilitation*.

Provident, I. & Joyce-Gaguzis, K. (2005). Brief Report–Creating an Occupational Therapy Level II Fieldwork Experience in a County Jail Setting. *American Journal of Occupational Therapy*, 59, 101-106.

Ravitch, D. & Viteritti, J. P. (Eds.). (2001). *Making good citizens: Education and civil society*. New York: Yale University Press.

Rice, R. E. (Fall, 2003). Rethinking scholarship & engagement: The struggle for new meanings. *Campus Compact Reader: Service Learning & Civic Education*, pp. 1-9.

Schön, D. (1983) *The reflective practitioner: How professionals think in action*. Basic Books.

Waddock, S. & Walsh, M. (1999). Paradigm shift: Toward a community-university community of practice. *The International Journal of Organizational Analysis*, 7 (3), 244-264.

ACADEMIC APPROACHES TO THE SCHOLARSHIP OF PRACTICE

Academic-Clinician Partnerships: A Model for Outcomes Research

Karen A. Stern, EdD, OT

SUMMARY. While practitioners are now asked to provide evidence that supports the services we deliver, there is little empirical evidence concerning occupational therapy interventions. Research by clinicians is limited, often due to a lack of time, institutional support and research skills. Establishing collaborative research relationships between faculty, clinicians, and graduate students has been suggested as a means of addressing these barriers. Implementation of a model teaming students

Karen A. Stern is Associate Professor and Chairperson, Kean University, Occupational Therapy Department, Union, NJ (E-mail: kstern@kean.edu).

The author thanks Rebecca Dutton, EdD, OT and Lynne Richard, MA, OT for their contributions and editorial guidance with this article. Portions of this article were presented at the American Occupational Therapy Association Annual Conference, Miami, Florida, May 2002.

[Haworth co-indexing entry note]: "Academic-Clinician Partnerships: A Model for Outcomes Research." Stern, Karen A. Co-published simultaneously in *Occupational Therapy in Health Care* (The Haworth Press, Inc.) Vol. 19, No. 1/2, 2005, pp. 95-106; and: *The Scholarship of Practice: Academic-Practice Collaborations for Promoting Occupational Therapy* (ed: Patricia Crist, and Gary Kielhofner) The Haworth Press, Inc., 2005, pp. 95-106. Single or multiple copies of this article are available for a fee from The Haworth Document Delivery Service [1-800-HAWORTH, 9:00 a.m. - 5:00 p.m. (EST). E-mail address: docdelivery@haworthpress.com].

Available online at http://www.haworthpress.com/web/OTHC
doi:10.1300/J003v19n01_07

with clinicians to conduct outcomes studies is described. The model will be illustrated using a case example of a collaborative research project evaluating the efficacy of a home management skills program for individuals with chronic mental illness. The benefits and challenges of the collaborative process will be described. *[Article copies available for a fee from The Haworth Document Delivery Service: 1-800-HAWORTH. E-mail address: <docdelivery@haworthpress.com> Website: <http://www.HaworthPress.com>* © *2005 by The Haworth Press, Inc. All rights reserved.]*

KEYWORDS. Outcomes research, collaborative partnerships, education, occupational therapy

Changes in the healthcare environment have significantly impacted upon the delivery of occupational therapy services. Practitioners are now asked to provide evidence that supports the services we deliver (Foto, 1996; Holm, 2000; Rogers & Holm, 1994). However, there is little empirical evidence concerning occupational therapy interventions (Ellenberg, 1996; Kielhofner, Hammel, Finlayson, Helfrich, & Taylor, 2004; Wood, 1998). The need to increase outcomes research to provide support for our practice is well documented. As Abreu, Peloquin and Ottenbacher (1998) state, "the achievement of competence in scientific inquiry and research is critical to the survival of the profession" (p. 751).

While there has been an increase in the number of clinicians engaging in research, most research is still conducted in academic settings. Several studies have explored clinician's attitudes towards research and research activities. It was found that clinicians who place a high value on research for the occupational therapy profession often cite a lack of time, institutional support and research skills as barriers to conducting research (Colborn, 1993; Cusick, Franklin, & Rotem, 1999; Cusick & Rotem, 1994; Stern, 2001; Taylor & Mitchell, 1990).

Establishing collaborative research relationships between faculty, clinicians, and graduate students has been suggested as a means of addressing the barriers faced by clinicians when undertaking a research project (Colborn, 1993). Several innovative academic-clinician partnerships have been described in the literature. Bloomer (1995) describes three models where there was collaboration between community clinicians and occupational therapy education programs in conducting research projects. At Dalhousie University, the curriculum includes a course where students design a research study, which is implemented during their final fieldwork experience. Faculty mentors and fieldwork supervisors work together to provide an integrative applied research experience for the students. A second model has students participate in a research application course, which follows a traditional research methods course. In the application course, students are assigned to work with a faculty member or clinician who is involved in applied research projects. Students assist in the research process. A third model offers the students an opportunity to develop a research project and integrate the project with Level II fieldwork experiences. Mercy College has established a collaborative research model involving faculty, clinicians, and students (Toglia, Golisz, Moulton & Daniel, 2001). Philips (2002) described how students collaborated together on a research project related to participation in a community wellness project.

The faculty at the University of Illinois at Chicago (UIC) have developed a strategy for developing scholars of practice based on social learning theory. Through the use of situated learning and cognitive apprenticeship strategies, the student's ability to link theory, research, and practice is facilitated. Students become participants in a community of scholars, where they have the opportunity to learn along with their advisors, peers, other faculty, clients, staff, practitioners and members of the community. This was achieved through the development of a "robust, scholarly community" in which the members of the community of scholars build upon each other's work. Students participate in one of the traditions of inquiry established within the occupational therapy department. These lines of inquiry involved community partnerships, with research questions generated from practice contexts (Braveman, Helfrich, & Fisher, 2001; Hammel, Finlayson, Kielhofner, Helfrich, & Peterson, 2001; Kielhofner, 2001).

The faculty at Kean University have developed a model for academic-clinician partnerships in response to the aforementioned issues, that incorporates aspects of existing collaborative partnership models. The development of the academic-clinician partnership model and its implementation will be described. A case example will be used to illustrate the academic-clinician partnership model.

THE ACADEMIC-CLINICIAN PARTNERSHIP MODEL

Development of the Model

In the mid 90's, the Kean University Occupational Therapy faculty began to develop a master's program to replace the existing certificate program and the first master's class was admitted in the fall of 1998. The faculty discussed at length the distinction between undergraduate and graduate education. Aside from the distinction in the level of critical thinking and academic rigor, the faculty focused on the development of a strong research component. This was essential with the implementation of the Standards for an Accredited Educational Program for the Occupational Therapist (ACOTE, 1999), which requires that all graduates be able to "provide evidence-based effective therapeutic intervention related to performance areas" (p. 579) and to "design and implement beginning level research studies" (p. 581). The initial program included a two-semester research course. To maximize use of faculty resources, students worked in small groups to develop and implement a research project.

The faculty wrestled with the issue of what can be done to develop the research skills of the students and provide a meaningful research experience for them. The goal was to provide a variety of research experiences to choose from, anywhere from developing individual research ideas, teaming with a faculty member in an ongoing project or possibly working collaboratively with clinicians on outcomes research.

The idea for collaborative research was shared with several clinicians who provide fieldwork experiences for our students. Based on several conversations with clinicians who were attempting to conduct outcomes research in their facilities, the need for assistance with this process became apparent. Clinicians cited the lack of time and skill as barriers to conducting outcomes research. We felt that we could help overcome the obstacles faced by the clinicians. We could provide student research teams to provide the manpower and research skills required to conduct the research. The clinician would provide the research question and the resources to collect the data, while the university provides the resources and technical support for the development of the research proposal, data collection and analysis and report of the research findings.

The development of the collaborative research model began with a review of existing models. Our model incorporated aspects of several existing collaborative partnership models (Bloomer, 1995; Braveman, Helfrich, & Fisher, 2001; Hammel et al., 2001; Toglia, Golisz, Moulton, & Daniel, 2001). In her description of three models of collaborative research partnerships, Bloomer (1995) described the essential characteristics shared by all of the models. These included: (1) an educational program that requires participation in research; (2) an active network of clinician and academicians committed to scientific inquiry,

(3) a desire on the part of these clinicians and academicians to further their own research activity, (4) a highly structured format to help ensure that each student's role in the research is a valuable learning experience and, if possible, a success oriented activity, if not in outcome, at least in process, and (5) an expectation of an end product (p. 208). Our collaborative research partnership embraces these characteristics. Consistent with the UIC scholarship of practice model, social learning theory is used as a framework for our approach to teaching research. "Knowledge is situated, being in part a product of the activity, context, and culture in which it is developed and used" (Brown, Collins, & Duguid, 1989, p. 32). Thus, providing students the opportunity to acquire and apply research skills in a meaningful context will facilitate understanding of the research process. The students are socialized into the role of researcher and scholar.

Structure of the Model

Students complete a two-semester sequence of research courses, which requires the students to plan and implement a research project. The first course is a traditional research methods course. During this course, the students are guided through the process of developing a research proposal. The second course provides students with the opportunity to implement the research project. Prior to the start of the research course sequence, proposed research topics are developed through collaboration of the faculty member(s) teaching the course sequence and the clinicians. At the beginning of the research methods course, students are presented with the available research topics and given an opportunity to select a topic that reflects their own interests as much as possible. This is essential, as it is important that the research be of interest to the student and also be relevant to current occupational therapy practice.

Once groups and topics are determined, the students, along with the faculty member and clinician, operationalize the research question. Each group is assigned a faculty mentor with expertise and/or research experience in the student's topic area. The students are mentored through the process of developing the research proposal, with ongoing input from the faculty and the clinician. At the end of the semester, the proposal is submitted to the university institutional research board (IRB) as well as the agency where the research will take place. Any required modifications are made at the beginning of the second course, prior to implementation.

During the second course, the students engage in the data collection and analysis process, and write a report of the results. Ongoing guidance from the faculty mentor, along with collaboration with the clinician facilitates the process. All students meet together once a week to discuss the status of their project and share their experiences with their peers and faculty mentors. Upon completion of the research report, students present their research studies to faculty members, students and clinicians involved with the project. Plans are made for presentation and/or publication of the research study.

IMPLEMENTATION OF THE ACADEMIC-CLINICIAN PARTNERSHIP MODEL: A CASE EXAMPLE

The evaluation of the efficacy of a new home management skills program in a community based consumer run program for individuals with chronic mental illness illustrates the implementation of the academic-clinician partnership model. The impetus for the first academic-clinician partnership was the development of a home management skills program for a consumer-run program for individuals with chronic mental illness by two graduate students as part of the requirements in their administration course. The associate director of the consumer-run program, an occupational therapist, decided to implement the program using agency staff and occupational therapy fieldwork II students to staff the program and asked for assistance with the evaluation of the efficacy of the program. Thus, the opportunity for the development of our academic-clinician partnerships was born.

Establishing the Collaborative Process

The faculty member responsible for teaching the research course sequence assumed the role of faculty mentor. Prior to the start of the semester, the faculty member met with the clinician to establish the groundwork for the research project. The clinician and faculty member established the distribution of responsibilities for the research project. The clinician would review the proposal and provide feedback about the methodology as it was developed, provide assistance with scheduling of data collection, and serve as contact person for all staff and clients involved with the process. The faculty member's role was to serve as research advisor, providing guidance through the entire planning and implementation process. The faculty member worked with the students in the development of the proposal and provided mentoring in the data collection and analysis process. This role delineation was important to establish before we could proceed any further and was critical to the success of the project.

Early in the spring semester, the faculty mentor and students established a timeline for the development of the research proposal. The research proposal was to be completed at the end of the spring semester. This allowed ample time to submit the proposal to the Kean University Institutional Research Board at the end of the spring semester and receive approval from the IRB, as well as the IRB of the clinical facility, before the implementation of the project during the fall semester.

Two meetings were scheduled with the clinician, one early in the semester, and one towards the end of the semester. During the first meeting with the clinician, the methodology used to evaluate program outcomes was established, as well as clarification of the roles and responsibilities of the faculty member, students and clinician. The students developed the proposal and instruments to be used, receiving feedback from the clinician and faculty member. As the proposal neared completion, the students and faculty member met once again with the clinician to ensure that there was agreement on the soundness of the research proposal.

When the students returned in the fall, a meeting was held with the clinician to establish a timeline for data collection. The students worked directly with the clinician to schedule interviews with staff and clients. An hour was set aside each week for the students and faculty member to meet on an as needed basis. The students were responsible for the data collection and data analysis process, with assistance from faculty members. In addition, the faculty member ensured that the students followed the established time line as best as possible.

At the conclusion of the project, the students presented their findings to the faculty, clinician, and other students in the occupational therapy program. Results of the project have been submitted for publication. The clinician received a copy of the final research report to share with her staff. The findings of the research project were used to enhance the home management program at the clinical facility.

Home Management Skills Program Evaluation Project

The purpose of the research project was to determine the effectiveness of the home management skills program. Eight staff members and seven residents agreed to participate in the study. Staff members were given a questionnaire designed to identify which home management skills were addressed during the implementation of the program. In addition, in-depth interviews of the staff members were conducted. The interview focused on the staff member's perception of the effectiveness of the program, identifying the strengths and limitations of the program, how the staff member implemented the program, what strategies were successful or needed modification and recommendations for the future.

The clients completed a questionnaire used to gather feedback about their participation in the program and their perception of the impact of the program on their home management skills. In addition, clients were interviewed to obtain information about the effectiveness of the program, the strengths and limitations of the program, helpfulness of the staff, and whether they felt that they acquired new skills. The students developed the questionnaires and interview questions, with input from the faculty member and clinician.

It was found that the most frequently addressed skills addressed were kitchen cleaning, vacuuming and kitchen appliance maintenance. Analysis of the staff interviews revealed four themes: importance of the program, motivational strategies utilized, program structure and difficulties encountered during program implementation. All staff members felt that the program was a necessary addition to the services provided to the clients, as many clients now residing in the community either were hospitalized for many years or cared for by family and lacked the skills necessary for independently living in the community. Motivating clients to participate in home management activities was a challenge and staff members devised individualized methods to motivate participation in the activities. Each staff member described their approach to structuring the program, using skills learned in their training, such as establishing a trusting relationship, providing graded structure, repetition and ongoing follow-up with the clients. Staff members described the difficulty with working with low functioning individuals and how difficult it was for the clients to make progress.

The clients reported feeling more confident about their home management skills as a result of participating in the program and were able to identify areas requiring further improvement. Three themes emerged from the interview data: staff support, helpful approaches utilized by staff, and carryover of newly learned skills. Staff support was essential for their success in learning new skills. The approaches used by staff to motivate and instruct the clients were viewed as helpful, and finally the support of staff was viewed as essential to maintaining the skills learned.

Overall, the staff and clients felt that the program was successful. A series of recommendations to enhance the program were made, such as consistent implementation and follow-up of clients. In addition, outcomes studies that include pre- and post-testing of the clients were strongly recommended. Due to time constraints, the structure of the program and staffing issues, it was not feasible to include these measures in this study.

Benefits and Challenges of the Collaborative Process

One of the most significant benefits of this research project was the learning opportunity provided to the students. They felt that participation in a research program in the clinical setting enhanced their learning and provided a meaningful experience for them. Along with developing research skills, the students developed an understanding of the positive aspects as well as the difficulties one encounters when conducting research in the clinical setting. Without the collaborative process, it is unlikely that a study of the effectiveness of the program would have been implemented. In this primarily consumer run organization, most staff members do not possess the research skills necessary to implement a research project.

The most significant challenge was the time commitment of the faculty member and staff members. The students had to be flexible and frequently adjust their timeline and schedule in accordance with the scheduling needs of the clinical site. In addition, the students were required to modify their methodology to accommodate the needs of the clients and the clinical program. For example, initially the students were to interview the clients. However, the staff felt that it would be more effective if they were to conduct the interviews. As they had an established relationship with the clients, it was more likely that the clients would agree to participate in the interview process. This in turn, added additional time constraints, as it took considerable time for staff to complete the interviews and the students had a very limited time allotted for completion of the data analysis.

Evaluation of the Academic-Clinician Partnership Model

Based on program evaluation data gathered upon completion of the research course sequence, it was determined that the changes to the research sequence were needed. The original research sequence consisted of two courses. The two-course sequence did not allow sufficient time to cover topics in the depth required at the graduate level as well as complete the research proposal. As a result, the research course sequence was expanded to a three-semester sequence of classes to allow for the time needed to facilitate development of the student's role as researcher and scholar.

Several limitations of the collaborative process were identified. The process is time consuming, faculty resources are limited and there are constraints placed on student's interaction with clients at the clinical sites. The faculty is currently evaluating the collaborative research process and identifying ways to reduce the demand on faculty time and resources, while maintaining a valuable research experience for the students.

Learning outcomes for the research courses were measured though a series of increasingly complex written assignments, culminating in a complete research report, as well as through examinations. Upon conclusion of the research project, a focus group with the students was held to discuss the process and outcomes of the courses. Results indicated that the students met and/or exceeded the stated learning objectives of the courses, despite the condensed nature of the research methods course. The students concurred with the faculty about the need for expansion of the research course sequence.

PLANS FOR THE FUTURE

The faculty is in the process of expanding the opportunities to institute the collaborative model of research. Discussions have taken place with several clinicians that have expressed an interest in this process. Establishing a line of research that can be continued each year by a new group of students is underway, based in part, on the UIC scholarship of practice model. Finally, the faculty is interested in evaluating the impact of the students' participation in the collaborative research projects on their subsequent involvement in research activities. This is a potential topic for student research in the future.

CONCLUSION

Stern (2001) found that there is little in the literature that describes how educators "actually translate their beliefs about the fundamental importance of research into educational practice. Occupational therapy educators have not articulated a range of strategies designed to help students become researchers" (p. 102). The establishment of the academic-clinician collaborative research projects provides a framework for socializing students into the role of researcher and consumer of research. Participation in the collaborative research projects provides students the opportunity to develop basic research skills, as well as reinforcing the importance of participating in research in their clinical practice.

Upon completion of the collaborative research project, the students discovered that they had the fundamental skills to conduct research and developed a better appreciation of their role as a researcher as an integral aspect of their professional life. In addition, clinicians benefited from the mentoring and support received through collaboration with an academic program. Finally, the academic-clinician partnerships made and will hopefully continue to contribute to the body of knowledge of the occupational therapy profession through the presentation and publication of the research findings. Overall, while requiring a considerable amount of work, this partnership was a win-win situation for all involved and the faculty looks forward to continuing with the collaborative process in the future.

REFERENCES

Abreu, B. C., Peloquin, S. M., & Ottenbacher, K. (1998). Competence in scientific inquiry and research. *American Journal of Occupational Therapy, 52,* 751-759.

Bloomer, J. S. (1995). Applied research during fieldwork: Interdisciplinary collaboration between universities and clinics. *American Journal of Occupational Therapy, 49,* 207-213.

Braveman, B. H., Helfrich, C. A., & Fisher, G. S. (2001). Developing and maintaining community partnerships within a scholarship of practice. *Occupational Therapy in Health Care, 15 (1/2),* 109-125.

Brown, J. S., Collins, A., & Duguid, P. (1989). Situated cognition and the culture of learning. *Educational Researcher, 18 (1),* 32-41.

Colborn, A. P. (1993). Combining practice and research. *American Journal of Occupational Therapy, 47,* 693-703.

Crepeau, E. B. (Ed.). (2001). *Research across the curriculum.* Bethesda, MD: American Occupational Therapy Foundation.

Cusick, A., Franklin, A., & Rotem, A. (1999). Meanings of "research" and "researcher": The clinician perspective. *Occupational Therapy Journal of Research, 19,* 101-125.

Cusick, A., & Rotem, A. (1994). Definitions of research by occupational therapy clinicians: An exploratory study. *Australian Occupational Therapy Journal, 41,* 99-114.

Ellenberg, D. B. (1996). Outcomes research: The history, debate and implications for the field of occupational therapy. *American Occupational Therapy Association, 50,* 435-441.

Foto, M. (1996). Outcome studies: The what, why, how, and when. *American Journal of Occupational Therapy, 50,* 87-88.

Hammel, J., Finlayson, M., Kielhofner, G., Helfrich, C. A., & Peterson, E. (2001). Educating scholars of practice: An approach to preparing tomorrow's researchers. *Occupational Therapy in Health Care, 15 (1/2),* pp. 157-176.

Holm, M. B. (2000). Our mandate for the new millennium: Evidence-based practice, 2000 Eleanor Clarke Slagle lecture. *American Journal of Occupational Therapy, 54,* 575-585.

Kielhofner, G. (2001). UIC's scholarship of practice. *OT Practice, 7 (1),* 11-12.

Kielhofner, G., Hammel, J., Finlayson, M., Helfrich. C., & Taylor, R. R. (2004). Documenting outcomes of occupational therapy: The center for outcomes research and education. *American Journal of Occupational Therapy, 58,* 15-23.

Phillips, I. (2002). Occupational therapy students explore an area for future practice in HIV/AIDS community wellness. *AIDS Patient Care and STDs, 16,* 147-149.

Rogers, J. C., & Holm, M. B. (1994). Nationally speaking: Accepting the challenge of outcome research: Examining the effectiveness of occupational therapy practice. *American Journal of Occupational Therapy, 48,* 871-876.

Stern, P. (2001). Occupational therapists and research: Lessons learned from a qualitative research course. *American Journal of Occupational Therapy, 55,* 102-105.

Taylor, E., & Mitchell. M. (1990). Research attitudes and activities of occupational therapy clinicians. *American Journal of Occupational Therapy, 44,* 350-355.

Toglia, J., Golisz, K., Moulton, H., & Daniel. S. (2001). Facilitating groups of students for research. In E. B. Crepeau (Ed.), *Research across the curriculum: A guide for occupational therapy educators.* Bethesda, MD: American Occupational Therapy Foundation.

Wood, W. (1998). It is jump time for occupational therapy. *American Occupational Therapy Association, 52,* 403-411.

Synthesizing Research, Education, and Practice According to the Scholarship of Practice Model: Two Faculty Examples

Renee R. Taylor, PhD
Gail Fisher, MPA, OTR/L
Gary Kielhofner, DrPH, OTR/L, FAOTA

SUMMARY. The Scholarship of Practice involves an ongoing, reflective discourse among the theoretical concepts of occupational therapy, the empirical verification of those concepts through research, and the application of those concepts in real-world clinical practice. This article illustrates how the Scholarship of Practice framework is applied by occupational therapy faculty members as a key aspect of their scholarly

---

Renee R. Taylor is Associate Professor, Gail Fisher is Clinical Associate Professor, and Gary Kielhofner is Professor, all at the University of Illinois at Chicago, Department of Occupational Therapy, Chicago, IL.

Address correspondence to: Renee R. Taylor, PhD, University of Illinois at Chicago, Department of Occupational Therapy, 1919 West Taylor Street (MC 811), Chicago, IL 60612 (E-mail: rtaylor@uic.edu).

Funding support for the research studies discussed in this paper was provided by National Institute on Disability and Rehabilitation Research Grant #: H133G010136 and by the National Institute of Child Health and Human Development and the Office of Research on Women's Health Grant #: R01 HD4330101A1.

[Haworth co-indexing entry note]: "Synthesizing Research, Education, and Practice According to the Scholarship of Practice Model: Two Faculty Examples." Taylor, Renee R., Gail Fisher, and Gary Kielhofner. Co-published simultaneously in *Occupational Therapy in Health Care* (The Haworth Press, Inc.) Vol. 19, No. 1/2, 2005, pp. 107-122; and: *The Scholarship of Practice: Academic-Practice Collaborations for Promoting Occupational Therapy* (ed: Patricia Crist, and Gary Kielhofner) The Haworth Press, Inc., 2005, pp. 107-122. Single or multiple copies of this article are available for a fee from The Haworth Document Delivery Service [1-800-HAWORTH, 9:00 a.m. - 5:00 p.m. (EST). E-mail address: docdelivery@haworthpress.com].

and teaching roles. Two distinct perspectives are provided–one describes the scholarship and teaching of a clinical-track faculty member and the other describes that of a research-track faculty member. Both examples illustrate how each faculty member's work involves an integration of teaching and advising, scholarship (i.e., developing occupational therapy theory and conducting research), and practice. In both cases, the faculty member uses the Scholarship of Practice approach to better understand the kinds of problems and needs of clients and the ways in which practitioners can use knowledge generated by theory and research to most effectively address them. In turn, each faculty member relies heavily on the feedback from students and practitioners regarding the outcomes of the practical application of the concepts offered by theory and research. This feedback is then utilized to revise and refine existing theory, generate new research questions, and ultimately inform best occupational therapy practice. Finally the process serves as an ideal context for teaching and advising. *[Article copies available for a fee from The Haworth Document Delivery Service: 1-800-HAWORTH. E-mail address: <docdelivery@haworthpress.com> Website: <http://www.HaworthPress.com> © 2005 by The Haworth Press, Inc. All rights reserved.]*

KEYWORDS. Scholarship of Practice, occupational therapy, education

Building a vision of scholarship that demonstrates real-world application of theory and research to practice is a challenge that occupational therapy educators must face (Kielhofner, 2005). A growing number of writers have examined this challenge and its importance to the field (Abreu, Peloquin & Ottenbacher, 1998; Christiansen, 1981; Hammel, 2000; Hammel, Finlayson, Kielhofner, Helfrich, & Peterson, 2002; Kielhofner, 2000; Kielhofner, 2005; Taylor, Braveman, & Forsyth, 2002). These writers share the observation that there is a disturbing gap between the propagation of increasingly numerous theoretical concepts in the field and the extent to which these concepts are actually applied in clinical practice settings. A similar inconsistency has been observed between the kinds of research studies conducted in academic settings and the actual questions and therapeutic approaches that practitioners see as relevant to clinical outcomes (Abreu, Peloquin, & Ottenbacher, 1998; Hammel et al., 2002; Kielhofner, in press). Approximately one decade ago, the concept of a Scholarship of Practice was developed at the University of Illinois (UIC) as a response to this challenge. A central aim of the Scholarship of Practice is to promote the formation of a cumulative body of occupational therapy knowledge that is empirically grounded and readily applied to practice in real-world clinical settings (Kielhofner & Crist, this issue; Kielhofner, Borell, & Tham, 2002; Kielhofner, 2002).

It calls for real-world application of ideas and evidence generated in the academic setting. The Scholarship of Practice requires a planned, structured, and synergistic approach to scholarship. Implementing it is a challenging task requiring a great deal of thought and planning to organize necessary resources. It also requires a strong investment in the aim of a scholarship of practice by individual faculty members. The fragmentation of education, faculty scholarship and practice exists because there are substantial organizational and logistic challenges to its implementation, which calls for an integration of one's educational, scholarly, and service missions.

Integrating the education of students, the conduct of scholarship, and involvement in service can occur in multiple ways. In our experience it works best when organized across an entire curriculum, as well as within a single faculty member's research laboratory or student advising team. Hammel and associates (2002) have described how the scholarship of practice serves as an underlying foundation of a comprehensive occupational therapy curriculum within the Department of Occupational Therapy at the University of Illinois (UIC). In this paper, we will focus on how individual faculty members can utilize the Scholarship of Practice as a personal framework. Specifically, we will describe how faculty members can integrate their research, service, student advising, and teaching responsibilities into a coherent vision of scholarship. Two examples will be presented. One example will be drawn from the work of a clinical-track faculty member and one was drawn from the work of a research-track faculty member.

THE SCHOLARSHIP OF PRACTICE

The Scholarship of Practice is a natural outgrowth of the heritage of the Department of Occupational Therapy at the University of Illinois (UIC). Under the direction of Beatrice D. Wade, the department was founded in 1943 on a model that integrated practice and education according to what was then known as the "Illinois Plan." According to this plan, students of occupational therapy were taught to apply theoretical principles of occupational therapy learned in the classroom to their actual clinical practice, which occurred down the street at the University of Illinois Hospital. Unique and unprecedented at the time, the same faculty members teaching classroom concepts served as the clinical educators and supervisors in the clinical setting. As a result of its history, the department has upheld its traditional value that concepts learned in classroom and practice settings should overlap and be mutually informative.

The notion of linking theory, research, and practice into a cohesive vision of scholarship is a contemporary offspring of the Illinois Plan. This notion developed into the Scholarship of Practice model a decade ago to identify a common vision for occupational therapy scholarship. A second influential underpinning of the Scholarship of Practice model is UIC's Great Cities mission (Perry, Alpern, Harnbleton, Manning, & Tanner, 2003). This mission promotes faculty and student engagement in applied research and service activities that support and empower individuals living in underserved, urban environments. Thus, the university favors engagement in research activities that are not only relevant to the immediate intrapersonal consequences of disability, but are also relevant to the secondary social and economic consequences of disability that are often heightened in resource-limited urban settings.

Today's vision of scholarship, the Scholarship of Practice (Kielhofner & Crist, this issue; Kielhofner, in press), involves an ongoing discourse between the theoretical concepts of occupational therapy, the empirical verification of those concepts through research, and the application of those concepts in real-world clinical practice. In turn, problems encountered in the everyday application of these concepts in practice then inform and raise additional questions to be addressed in the future development and refinement of new and existing theoretical concepts, and new research hypotheses. This process is depicted in Figure 1.

The aim of these efforts is to better understand the kinds of problems and needs addressed by occupational therapy and the ways in which the field can most effectively address them. This aim reflects the belief that science and scholarship in occupational therapy should proceed in the interest of solving real practice problems and that occupational therapy scholars should give intellectual priority articulating occupational problems and developing workable solutions.

The Approach to Scholarship at UIC. We envision that all scholarship in the department will generate knowledge to enhance the process and outcomes of practice. Scholarship may embrace efforts to generate new knowledge through research. It may also encompass development

FIGURE 1. A Scholarship of Practice

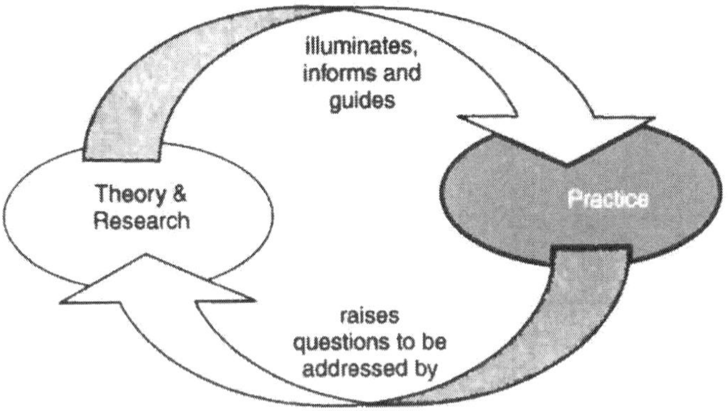

efforts that involve applications of theory and empirical findings through critical and reflective generation and refinement of practice resources. Faculty scholarship (both research and development) in the department is diverse, and includes clarifying the occupational strengths and challenges of certain populations, identifying service needs, testing theory from models of practice, creating and refining assessments and intervention strategies, examining the influence of culture, economics, policy and other contextual factors on practice, and determining how to best achieve positive outcomes of therapy.

Approach to Education. At UIC a fundamental idea is that students, who are learning to become practitioners or who are advancing their knowledge about practice, best learn by actively engaging the scholarly process that examines and develops knowledge and tools for practice. This strategy reflects concepts of social learning theory and employs situated learning approaches that involve students as apprentices in an ongoing community of scholars (Hammel et al., 2002). Our aim for our students is that they learn how knowledge is applied, value processes that lead to the refinement of knowledge and its application in practice. For the individual faculty member, this means that a significant portion of one's educational effort (teaching courses, advising student projects and research) is integrated into and helps to advance one's ongoing scholarship.

Approach to Service. As noted earlier the Great Cities commitment (Perry et al., 2003) at UIC strongly influences our vision that we have a mission to address problems in the urban context. At UIC this means that each faculty member identifies settings and/or populations that are the target of one's service efforts. Service generally includes not only efforts to create and test interventions at a particular site or with a particular population, but also synergistic activities such as service on the agency board, consulting to the agency, and developing collaborative relationships with the agency that involve other departmental personnel.

Integrating Scholarship, Education and Service. The Scholarship of Practice means that we integrate our educational, practice and research efforts. This means that faculty members each develop an individual approach to bringing these elements together. The following are two examples of how faculty members incorporate their research into a vision of scholarship that is grounded in the Scholarship of Practice. In the first example, a clinical faculty member works with students to develop and refine theory-based assessments and interventions for a community agency serving adults with intellectual/developmental disabilities. The second example illustrates how a research faculty member's vision of scholarship is actualized through involvement with students in two federally-funded research studies.

EXAMPLE FROM A CLINICAL TRACK FACULTY MEMBER

As a clinical associate professor, the second author's role includes responsibilities in teaching, supervision of master's projects, and collaborative research with research track faculty members. Linking these role components together under the umbrella of the Scholarship of Practice model requires a synergy that allows each component to be linked to and to build on the others. One mode of integrating several role components is the community practicum sequence at UIC. This situated learning experience is comprised of a three-course sequence, and requires all professional master's students to spend an average of three hours per week at the same community agency for over a year. Students are co-supervised by their faculty liaison, who is typically their faculty advisor, and a community site supervisor. The practicum is carried out in the context of the urban (Great Cities) mission at UIC, and it prepares students to work with multiethnic, underserved populations residing in the city of Chicago. It also provides an opportunity for faculty to develop a relationship with a community agency that can support the development of scholarship in addition to training students. The building and maintenance of this relationship has been described previously (Braveman, Helfrich, & Fisher, 2001).

The second author developed a relationship with the adult program division at El Valor, an agency on the West side of Chicago serving primarily Hispanic adults with intellectual disabilities. El Valor's mission is to ". . . explore and develop opportunities that strengthen skills, knowledge and confidence in a linguistically and culturally supportive setting" (El Valor, 2003). The agency runs a day program for 70 individuals focused on vocational development and life enrichment, and six residential homes. Community practicum students are placed in either the day program or one of the group homes.

As students completed their practicum, two unmet needs became apparent to the students and the second author, who served as their faculty liaison and also their master's final project advisor. These two needs provided the impetus for the development of two projects that exemplify the scholarship of practice. The first project focused on the need for training and support for the staff at El Valor, particularly in planning, implementing, and evaluating group activities. This led to the development of a framework for staff development, using the Model of Human Occupation (Kielhofner, 2002). The second project grew out of a desire to make the residential home environment more supportive of occupational role development and quality of life for the residents. This led to the development of the *Residential Environment Impact Survey* (Fisher, Arriaga, Less, & Lee, 2003), an assessment and consulting tool also based on the Model of Human Occupation. Initially, this work took the form of final master's projects that were completed by teams of two students working with the second author. This area of scholarship has continued to be developed through subsequent student projects and the second author's efforts.

The two projects began with a thorough look at the literature to ascertain what studies were relevant to the development of these two new intervention tools. The new edition of the Model of Human Occupation was also used to provide the theoretical underpinning for these projects, and relevant assessments based on the Model were analyzed. This is one of the hallmarks of the scholarship of practice model. Practice innovations are based on theory and research. The other side of the coin is for practice to inform theory and research. This question was integrated into this scholarly work from the beginning: What have we learned from creating and using these instruments that will make the theory better, and will guide future research?

Creating the Staff Development Framework. Using the Model of Human Occupation and existing assessments as the base, the student teams, in collaboration with the second author, developed new assessments and intervention frameworks. These are non-standardized assessments that are used to guide a consultative intervention. For the staff development project, it was determined that baseline assessments were needed to get a picture of a staff member's interests, their view of what they did well, what they wanted to improve on, and how well the environment supported their efforts. A modification was done of the Occupational Self-Assessment © (Baron, Kielhofner, Goldhammer, & Wolenski, 1999), which is a tool used by occupational therapists with patients/clients to assist in determining their goals and self-perception of strengths and areas for improvement. With permission, the same format was used to develop a Staff Development Self-Assessment (Fisher, Nikiforos, & Cohen, 2002), but the items were revised to reflect the focus on the staff member's capability in setting appropriate goals, planning and leading groups, determining the right amount of support needed for the clients, locating resources, documenting outcomes, etc. Since the items are self-rated on adequacy of performance as well as importance, this provides a basis for goals for staff development that are determined by the staff member and the occupational therapist collaboratively. The Interest Checklist (Heasman, 2002) was also adapted to focus on the interests of the staff member, and whether they were interested in developing group activities for clients based on those interests (Fisher, Nikiforos & Cohen, 2002). Lastly, an interview was devised which was modeled on the Occupational Performance History Interview © (Kielhofner, Mallinson, Crawford, Nowak, Rigby, Henry, & Walens, 1997), but which focused on the roles of the staff member and their satisfaction and self-efficacy.

A review of the literature in related fields assisted in shaping the intervention phase of this project. Based on the Model of Human Occupation and the research in the field of staff training and development, an intervention program was developed that provided the staff member with a coach for several weeks to address up to five goals identified in the self-assessment phase.

This assessment and intervention framework for staff development was pilot tested with two staff members. The impact was measured through observations, a final interview, and supervisor feedback. Assessment tools and intervention strategies were then refined and presented to the administration of El Valor. This innovative use of the Model of Human Occupation was also shared with Kielhofner and others in the field of developmental disabilities to illustrate an application of the MOHO for staff development in addition to its use with patients/clients.

Developing the Residential Environment Impact Scale. The development of the Residential Environment Impact Survey (REIS) (Fisher, Arriaga, Less, & Lee, 2003) proceeded along a similar path of reviewing relevant theories, research and other assessments, developing the survey instrument, pilot testing it, refining it, and presenting results to the agency. The Model of Human Occupation (MOHO) was very relevant to the intended use of the survey, and the MOHO's conceptualization of environment provided a framework for organizing the instrument. Using the MOHO constructs of space, objects, occupational forms, and social groups for the REIS allowed data collection in a systematic way that linked back to the theory and how it has been applied in other environmental interventions.

Informing Theory and Research. As the REIS was designed and implemented, it became clear that the environment section of the MOHO did not fully account for certain important elements. For example, time dimensions of the group home were important aspects of the environment, but were not emphasized in the MOHO. Also, the focus of the environment section of the MOHO is on how the environment influences what we choose to do, and what factors in the environment influence occupation (Kielhofner, 2002). A fuller description would address how the environment is shaped by the actions of the people who are part of the environment, and how it is possible to influence occupational functioning by modifying the environment. This insight will influence revisions to the environmental aspect of MOHO in the future.

How can these two projects shape research in this neglected area of occupational therapy practice? The second author will continue to test and refine these instruments, in collaboration with future community practicum students and final project advisees. In addition, both of these projects are now being used in research conducted by other occupational therapists. Through a developmental disabilities list serve, an occupational therapist in another state found out about the staff development framework and will be using it in a study he designed to meet his post-professional degree thesis requirements, applying it with the staff at a large state-run residential facility. The Residential Environment Impact Survey is now being used as a tool in a newly funded study of community participation of adults with intellectual disabilities who are aging. The second author will be participating in that project as a research collaborator.

Future Directions. Dissemination of both tools will be accomplished in the near future, as manuals will be created and available for purchase from the Model of Human Occupation Clearinghouse (moho@uic.edu).

They will also be presented at national conferences and through peer-reviewed publications (Fisher, 2004, September). The students who contributed will be co-authors on the manuals.

Responsibilities for supervising students doing their community practicum at El Valor opened the door for the second author to develop a line of scholarship to address unmet needs within the agency. The scholarship of practice model provided a framework that guided the development of these clinical innovations, which can be used by occupational therapists practicing with a variety of populations. In the future, these application tools will shape theory development and research to assist people with disabilities in maximizing their participation in home and community environments.

EXAMPLE FROM A RESEARCH-TRACK FACULTY MEMBER

As a tenured associate professor at the University of Illinois at Chicago, the first author's central role revolves around conducting funded research studies that focus on fatigue as a physical, psychological, and social phenomenon. Other responsibilities all relate directly to this area of research, and they include teaching, serving the academic and broader urban communities, and advising/supervising students and grant staff members. In addition, the first author has a private psychotherapy practice serving individuals with fatigue, and this practice experience contributes to her knowledge and understanding of individuals with fatigue. It also contributes to her practical and conceptual understanding of the therapeutic use of self, which has become a secondary area of scholarship which will also be discussed below.

The first author has used a wide range of theoretical and methodological approaches to study fatigue. The first author's theoretical orientation is best characterized as an integrative approach that draws upon knowledge and theoretical models from the fields of psychology, medicine, public health, disability studies, and occupational therapy. Methodologically, the first author uses basic science approaches to investigate the etiology and epidemiology of unexplained fatigue syndromes, such as chronic fatigue syndrome, and applied research approaches to develop and evaluate community-based rehabilitation programs for individuals with these conditions.

Briefly, chronic fatigue syndrome (CFS) is a baffling condition with no known, singular cause and cure that has found to be consistent across samples (Friedberg & Jason, 1998). It is characterized by unexplained, debilitating fatigue and a number of physical and cognitive symptoms. When the first author began studying CFS, it was relatively new to the scientific and practice communities. As such, very little was known regarding diagnostic criteria, etiology, epidemiology, functional consequences, treatment, and prognosis. Despite recent advances in all of these areas, much remains to be learned about this condition in each of these domains. Researching CFS during a critical period of rapid scientific growth has enabled the first author and her research/student advising team to contribute to the increased understanding of CFS in range of areas that have included diagnostics and assessment, epidemiology, social issues, and program development.

When applying the Scholarship of Practice model in everyday work, the first author relies on the mentoring model of training in the Department of Occupational Therapy at the University of Illinois at Chicago (Hammel et al., 2002). It is also one that is commonly used in the field of psychology, and it is the model according to which the first author received training in graduate school. A mentoring model of training means that the first author's advisees all focus on unexplained fatigue syndromes as their topical area for a master's project or thesis. To prepare them to work in this area, they elect the first author's course, "Fatiguing Conditions and Disability." In addition, most of her advisees are funded by one of the first author's grants and thus have the opportunity to work as a research assistant.

As an educator the first author relies upon her focused vision of scholarship as an overarching framework to guide the planning and implementation of research and practice activities. The everyday tasks of the research study at hand become the pragmatic tools for teaching and learning. Taken together, a focused vision of scholarship and specific research project tasks immerse students in an intellectual atmosphere that allows for a reciprocal educational experience for both the faculty member and students.

A major facet of the first author's scholarship includes efforts to promote knowledge and understanding of the cause, nature, and treatment of unexplained fatigue syndromes. Two specific research studies will be presented to illustrate how the first author integrates research, education, and clinical practice with students. Currently, students in the research lab are working on a five-year study of the etiology and epidemiology of post-infectious fatigue in adolescents. This study, "A Prospective Study of Chronic Fatigue Syndrome in Adolescents," is co-funded by the National Institutes of Child Health and Human Development and the Office of Research on Women's Health. Its central aim is to identify the predictors of post-infectious fatigue syndromes that follow an acute onset of infectious mononucleosis. In addition, the study aims to estimate the prevalence of adolescents that develop a post-infectious fatigue syndrome following mononucleosis. It aims to compare the adolescents with post-infectious fatigue syndromes with those that recover from mononucleosis normally in terms of behavioral, functional, psychosocial, and physiological variables.

In the elective class, Fatiguing Conditions and Disability, students learn about the theoretical models that drive the assessments that are being used in this study. Specifically, they learn to apply a biopsychosocial model to understanding the multifaceted nature of post-infectious fatigue. In addition, students learn to use the Model of Human Occupation to guide their understanding of the functional and occupational outcomes of fatigue. In the research lab, they learn to administer a number of assessments, each of which reflects either an aspect of the biopsychosocial model, or aspects of the Model of Human Occupation. Students working as research assistants in the lab are also required to establish and maintain relationships with the physicians that are involved in the study. Direct contact with the adolescent research subjects and the participating physicians allows students to develop their diagnostic and assessment skills, learn about the operations of a research study, and gain exposure to relationship-building within a multi-disciplinary health care team.

At the same time, students learn to critically evaluate rehabilitation programs that have been developed to empower individuals with fatigue. Initially, they learn these skills in the Fatiguing Conditions and Disability course through reading, discussion, and assignments that allow for understanding and critical thinking about current research studies and review articles that summarize the state of the science with respect to rehabilitation approaches for individuals with fatigue. They are then encouraged to apply their classroom learning to the development of a master's thesis or project that promotes further understanding of the quality and efficacy of various approaches to rehabilitation. Each thesis a student writes must be grounded in the given theory that underlies the study of a given outcome. Thus, students have the opportunity to choose and learn about a number of theories that range from empowerment theory (Rappaport, 1994) to conservation of resources theory (Hobfoll, 1998).

The first author recently finished implementing a three-year study that involved the development and evaluation of a community-based rehabilitation program for individuals with CFS. This study, "A Field-Initiated Research Project to Determine the Effectiveness of a Capacity-Building Program for Individuals with Chronic Fatigue Syndrome," was funded by the U.S. Department of Education, National Institute on Disability and Rehabilitation Research. This randomized clinical trial (Taylor, 2004) evaluated the effectiveness of a 12-month, participatory rehabilitation program. The contents of this program were shaped by direct input from individuals with chronic fatigue syndrome, and they were also influenced by the first author's experience treating clients with chronic fatigue syndrome in clinical practice. A number of outcomes that are directly relevant to practice were measured including functional capacity, coping, goal attainment, quality of life, resource acquisition, service utilization, coping, and illness severity, among others. Students who are interested in completing master's theses have the opportunity to select an area of interest within our existing database, develop a research hypothesis about a particular baseline variable or study outcome, and evaluate that hypothesis using statistical analyses. In addition to these outcomes, a byproduct of the program was the development of a program curriculum and a resource directory, both of which are available online *http://www.ahs.uic.edu/ahs/files/ot/bookler/CFS_ Website/index.htm* for use by occupational therapists in clinical practice.

Having two studies, a recently completed outcomes study and a beginning epidemiological study, is convenient because the recently completed study provides a database of outcomes for students to examine for their theses, while the study that is just beginning provides them with practice and supervision in study implementation, data collection and assessment skills. Because occupational therapy for individuals with chronic fatigue syndrome is a relatively new practice area, articles from the outcomes study that students co-author may be particularly important in informing occupational therapy practice with this population. In addition to these studies, our service relationships with community-based organizations that empower and advocate for individuals with unexplained fatigue syndromes have served to educate the first author and her students about the lived experiences and resource needs of a wider range of individuals with fatigue living in the community. Individuals in these community-based organizations have been instrumental in the planning and implementation of each of the first author's research studies. In addition, the first author's ongoing experience in clinical practice with clients with chronic fatigue syndrome has influenced the development of each of these studies and it has also influenced what she conveys to students in the classroom about individuals living with fatiguing illness.

A second facet of the first author's scholarship is just emerging, but also uses the scholarship of practice approach. As a clinical psychologist, the first author spent a great deal of time providing consultation to occupational therapists in clinical practice prior to entering the field in an academic capacity. As a result of these experiences, the first author has observed that the occupational therapy literature lacks a clearly articulated model of the role, mechanisms and processes underlying the therapeutic use of self in occupational therapy. In contrast there is a relatively well developed literature on the therapeutic relationship and the therapeutic use of self in psychology. Thus, the first author is in the process of developing a model of the therapeutic use of self in occupational therapy.

In accord with the Scholarship of Practice, development of this theoretical model will be, in part, based on the first author's prior experiences in clinical practice with occupational therapists. The model is being developed based on observations and input from occupational therapists currently in clinical practice. These practitioners are being interviewed and observed in interaction with their clients within the U.S. and internationally. Findings from these interviews will be mapped onto the model and published in book and article forms. Occupational therapy students are currently involved in gathering literature to support the development of this model and in co-developing a questionnaire with the first author that will evaluate the state of the field in terms of practitioners' knowledge and use of self in their interactions with clients.

CONCLUSION

In summary, the Scholarship of Practice involves an ongoing, reflective discourse between the theoretical concepts of occupational therapy, the empirical verification of those concepts through research, and the application of those concepts in real-world clinical practice. According to this framework, problems and successes that arise in the everyday application of theoretical concepts in practice are then noted and communicated back to the theorist. These lessons from practice inform and raise additional questions to be addressed in the future development and refinement of new and existing theoretical concepts. These concepts are then refined and re-examined in new and ongoing research studies.

The ultimate goal of the Scholarship of Practice is to better understand the kinds of problems and needs addressed by occupational therapy and the ways in which educators, theorists, researchers, and practitioners can most effectively address them. This aim reflects the belief that research and scholarship in occupational therapy should proceed in the interest of solving applied practice problems. In this vein, the Scholarship of Practice holds that occupational therapy scholars should give intellectual priority to elucidating occupational problems and developing workable solutions.

Educating students, building a tradition of independent scholarship, consulting with community-based organizations, and contributing to best occupational therapy practice are among the essential job tasks for occupational therapy faculty. The Scholarship of Practice is one means by which these tasks can be accomplished in a planned, focused, and practice-relevant way. Two distinct perspectives were provided on how a progressive dialectic between theory, research, education and practice can be created as part of the individual scholarship of faculty members. One example described the scholarship of a clinical-track faculty member and a second example described that of a research-track faculty member. Common to both perspectives is the importance of a focused vision of scholarship. Both faculty members selected a single clinical population (one selected people with intellectual disabilities and the other selected people with chronic fatigue syndrome) and each of them spent years developing knowledge and experience with that population. Sustaining focus on a single clinical problem enabled them to become conversant in the theoretical perspectives, relevant research, and existing practices used by occupational therapists in clinical practice. This focus, in combination with a respect for existing occupational therapy theory and knowledge, a trust in scientific empiricism, and most importantly, a valuing of feedback from clients, practitioners, and students, are the essential ingredients in building one's personal scholarship around a Scholarship of Practice framework.

REFERENCES

Abreu, B. C., Peloquin, S. M., & Ottenbacher, K. (1998). Competence in scientific inquiry and research. *The American Journal of Occupational Therapy, 52* (9), 751-759.

Baron, K., Kielhofner, G., Goldhammer, T., & Wolenski, J. (1999). *The Occupational Self Assessment* © University of Illinois, Model of Human Occupation Clearinghouse.

Braveman, B. H., Helfrich, C. A., Fisher, G. S. (2001). Developing and maintaining community partnerships within a scholarship of practice. *Occupational Therapy in Health Care,* 15 (1/2): 109-125.

Christiansen, C. (1981). Toward revolution of crisis: Research requisites in occupational therapy. *The Occupational Therapy Journal of Research, 1,* 115-124.

El Valor (2002). Program Management Reports 2002/2003. Unpublished report.

Fisher, G. S. (2004, September). The Residential Environment Impact Survey. *AOTA Developmental Disabilities: Special Interest Section Quarterly,* 27(3), 1-4.

Fisher, G. S., Arriaga, P., Less, C., & Lee, J. (2003). Residential Environment Impact Survey, Version 1.3. Unpublished instrument.

Fisher, G. S., Cohen, A., & Nikiforos, M. (2002). Interest Checklist for Staff Development. Unpublished instrument.

Fisher, G. S., Nikiforos, M., & Cohen, A. (2002). Staff Development Self-Assessment. Unpublished instrument.

Friedberg, F., & Jason, L. A. (1998). *Understanding Chronic Fatigue Syndrome.* American Psychological Association: Washington, DC.

Hammel, J., Finlayson, M., Kielhofner, G., Helfrich, C., & Peterson, E. (2002). Educating scholars of practice: An approach to preparing tomorrow's researchers. *Occupational Therapy in Health Care, 15 (1/2),* 157-176.

Hammel, J. (2000). Linking ICIDH-2 and OT theory to everyday practice. *Annual Illinois OT Association Conference,* Galena, IL, Oct. 31, 2000.

Heasman, D. (2002). Interest Checklist-UK version. Unpublished instrument.

Hobfoll, S. E. (1998). Stress, Culture, and Community: The Psychology and Philosophy of Stress. Personal communication. Plenum Press, NY.

Kielhofner, G. (2005). *Scholarship and Practice: Bridging the Divide. American Journal of Occupational Therapy.*

Kielhofner, G. (2002). *A Model of Human Occupation: Theory and Application* (3rd ed.). Baltimore: Williams & Wilkins.

Kielhofner, G. (2000). *A scholarship of practice: How knowledge development can best serve practice in the new millennium.* Keynote Address. British Occupational Therapy Annual Conference, Keele, England, July 18, 2000.

Kielhofner, G., Mallinson, T., Crawford, C., Nowak, M., Rigby, M., Henry, A., & Walens, D. (1997). *A User's Guide to the Occupational Performance History Interview-II* © University of Illinois, Model of Human Occupation Clearinghouse.

Kielhofner, G., Borell, L., & Tham, K. (2002). Preparing scholars of practice around the world. *OT Practice, 7 (6),* 13-14.

Kielhofner, G. (2002). UIC's scholarship of practice. *OT Practice, 7 (1),* 11-12.

Perry, D. C., Alpern, L., Hambleton, R., Manning, S., & Tanner, M. (2003). Great Cities Institute 2002-2003 Annual Report. Retrieved from the world wide web on March 29, 2004 at *www.greatcities.uic.*

Rappaport, J. (1994). Empowerment as a guide to doing research: Diversity as a positive value. In E. J. Trickett, R. J. Watts et al. (Eds.), *Human diversity: Perspectives on people in context.* San Francisco, CA: Jossey-Bass Inc.

Taylor, R. R., Braveman, B., & Forsyth, K. (2002). Occupational science and the scholarship of practice: Implications for practitioners. *New Zealand Journal of Occupational Therapy, 49,* 37-40.

Taylor, R. R. (2004). Quality of Life and Symptom Severity for Individuals with Chronic Fatigue Syndrome: Findings from a Randomized Clinical Trial. *American Journal of Occupational Therapy, 58,* 35-43.

A Collaborative Scholarly Project: Constraint-Induced Movement Therapy

Jan Stube, PhD, OTR/L, BCN

SUMMARY. This paper describes the phases of a scholarly project process within one occupational therapy (OT) professional program. Using the example of a scholarly project on constraint-induced movement therapy, the collective endeavor among two OT graduate students, a faculty advisor, and two occupational therapists is demonstrated. The process leading toward a clinically-relevant outcome provided benefits to all collaborators. The students experienced evidence-based scholarship firsthand, while the advisor and practitioners experienced the rewards of shaping a clinically useful product and received outcomes research assistance. The description of this scholarly project process serves as a model for future scholarly collaboration among graduate students, practitioners, and faculty members. *[Article copies available for a fee from The Haworth Document Delivery Service: 1-800-HAWORTH. E-mail address: <docdelivery@haworthpress.com> Website: <http://www.HaworthPress.com> © 2005 by The Haworth Press, Inc. All rights reserved.]*

Jan Stube is Assistant Professor, Department of Occupational Therapy, School of Medicine and Health Sciences, University of North Dakota, Grand Forks, ND 58202-7126 (E-mail: jstube@medicine.nodak.edu).

The author wishes to acknowledge Laura Beach, MOT, and Margo Iverson, MOT, for their creative and scholarly approach to their OT education, and Jane Loscheider, OTR, and Marsha Waind, OTR, CHT, for their invaluable advice in the development of this scholarly project outcome.

[Haworth co-indexing entry note]: "A Collaborative Scholarly Project: Constraint-Induced Movement Therapy." Stube, Jan. Co-published simultaneously in *Occupational Therapy in Health Care* (The Haworth Press, Inc.) Vol. 19, No. 1/2, 2005. pp. 123-133; and: *The Scholarship of Practice: Academic-Practice Collaborations for Promoting Occupational Therapy* (ed: Patricia Crist, and Gary Kielhofner) The Haworth Press, Inc., 2005. pp. 123-133. Single or multiple copies of this article are available for a fee from The Haworth Document Delivery Service [1-800-HAWORTH, 9:00 a.m. - 5:00 p.m. (EST). E-mail address: docdelivery@haworthpress.com].

doi:10.1300/J003v19n01_09

KEYWORDS. Scholarly project, occupational therapy, higher education

INTRODUCTION

Scholarship, as defined in higher educational circles, takes many forms and serves to embody lifelong learning. As proposed by Boyer (1990) and represented within an American Occupational Therapy Association Commission on Education (2003) concept paper, scholarship includes four overlapping forms: discovery, integration, application, and teaching. Scholarship, particularly through its discovery, integration, and application forms, is likely to uncover linkages and to advance a professional body of knowledge (Glassick, Huber, & Maeroff, 1997). As such, a scholarly project is one method for demonstration of clinical perspective and an integral understanding of a clinical practice topic for partial completion of a professional master's degree in occupational therapy. The purpose of this paper is to describe the scholarly project process at the University of North Dakota through one example of a scholarly project topic, constraint-induced movement therapy (CIMT). Through the description of this scholarly project process and example, the collaborative partnerships among occupational therapy (OT) graduate students, practitioners and faculty are illustrated, along with the benefits derived from the process for clinical practice.

BACKGROUND FOR COLLABORATIVE SCHOLARSHIP

To what extent does collaborative scholarship among professionals in occupational therapy prove critical to the advancement of our profession? Contributing to an evolving understanding of scholarship within practice, the health sciences literature details many collective benefits of collaborative research and other scholarly endeavors among practitioners, faculty members, and/or students. The benefits include: keeping clinical knowledge up-to-date, providing variety within the work role, maintenance of good working relationships, deliberate and deeper clinical reflection, an infusion of motivation and creativity, assistance for outcomes research, and students as part of the evidence-seeking and communication processes alongside professional role models (Bowman & Llewellyn, 2002; Colborn, 1993; Hague & Snyder, 1991; Hammel, Finlayson, Kielhofner, Helfrich, & Peterson, 2001; Mostrom, Capehart, Epstein, Woods-Reynolds, & Triezenberg, 1999; Rebovich, Wodarski,

Hurley, Rasor-Greenhalgh, & Stombaugh, 1994; Selker, 1994; Seymour, Kinn, & Sutherland, 2003; Williams, Bornor, & Law, 1989). These benefits embody the scholarship experience envisioned for our students by the occupational therapy faculty at the University of North Dakota (UND). As an established, accredited occupational therapy program yet with a newly developed professional master's degree, the faculty wanted to continue the rich history of community collaboration, while adding an evidence-based scholarly experience for students to deepen their understanding and connectedness to professional practice.

The occupational therapy curriculum at the University of North Dakota (UND) incorporates the theory of Occupational Adaptation, thus recognizing the central concepts of adaptive response to occupational challenges within the occupational environment of professional education (Schkade & Schultz, 1992; Schultz, 2000; Schultz & Schkade, 1992). To obtain the degree of master of occupational therapy (MOT) at UND, a scholarly project is designed by the student to promote not only the individual demonstration of mastering a subject using a scholarly inquiry process, but also to involve a professional partnership with an academic advisor and, likely, another OT student or OT practitioner(s). The scholarly project serves as the final academic challenge for a student within the MOT program at UND.

THE SCHOLARLY PROJECT PROCESS

The scholarly project at the Department of Occupational Therapy at UND is defined as "a collaborative investigation of a relevant professional topic and production of a scholarly report with approval of the major faculty advisor" (2002, p. 17). The scholarly project is written by the student(s) in formal chapter format, similar to a thesis. A full investigation of the available literature on the topic is conducted. A review of the literature is written by the student(s) and discussed with the OT advisor. To this extent, the scholarly project process resembles other graduate-level work, such as a thesis or independent study (Jenkins, Price, & Straker, 1998). Differentiating a scholarly project from a thesis is the scholarly project product. The scholarly project product may take a variety of forms (e.g., a practice topic education manual or a protocol for a practice technique) yet must prove to be an addition to existing OT practice. This product is either included within the scholarly project report itself or included as an appendix or separate document. Students may work in a two-person partnership to accomplish the scholarly project mission; however, each person must demonstrate a significant contribution toward the end-product. Although the intent of the scholarly project process is ultimately the creation of a scholarly project product linked to occupational therapy practice, the overall process as well as the product are both viewed as beneficial to the student's professional development.

The scholarly project process at UND begins with an idea from occupational therapy practice and the MOT student (i.e., phase 1), leading to the implementation of a clinically useful product developed through the scholarly project process (i.e., the final phase 4). The scholarly project process is presented in Table 1 which includes key inquiry to be addressed at each phase in order to help the student move forward. At phase 1, the initial scholarly project idea emanates from an aspect of occupational therapy practice: the literature and/or the practitioner influence. We find that the inclusion of occupational therapy practitioners as guest speakers within our curriculum serves as a stimulus for the students' interest in clinical topics for further study. In phase 2, after the idea has been discussed and initially developed by the student(s) with the faculty advisor, a "clinical practice checkpoint" is initiated by the student-advisor team to verify the idea and scholarly project product development with an OT practitioner for its clinical efficacy. The OT practitioner expert is suggested by the advisor, based upon knowledge of regional practitioners and their practice characteristics. At phase 1 or 2, the academic advisor initiates the Institutional Review Board approval process, as appropriate.

At phase 3, the student-advisor team initiates another meeting with the OT practitioner expert as a "clinical practice critique" of the scholarly project product. At this time, the product is enhanced or improved by the collaborative discussion as the student(s) finalize/s the product development and scholarly project report. At the completion of phase 3, the scholarly project overview is presented by the student(s) to fellow MOT students and occupational therapy faculty, and the product is presented to the practitioner expert for clinical implementation. The completion of phase 3 is also the point of graduation and entry into the world of clinical practice in occupational therapy.

Phase 4 signals the clinical implementation phase, whereby the practitioner may choose to use the product developed by the MOT student(s). The MOT students (now graduates) may use the product to promote their employability in job seeking or within their employment practice settings, thus extending the reach of the product implementation. At phase 4, the newly matriculated MOT practitioner, the higher education advisor, and the practitioner expert may voluntarily elect to

TABLE 1. Summary of the Scholarly Project Process

Phases of the Scholarly Project	Key Inquiry
1. **The Idea:** Clinical Practice Infusion	• Does the scholarly project idea emanate from OT practice and/or the practice literature? • How will the scholarly project idea contribute to the OT process or profession? • Does the scholarly project idea hold personal meaning and promote active involvement for the student?

2. **Development of the Idea:** Clinical Practice "Check-Point"	• What OT theoretical framework guides the development of the scholarly project idea?
	• How is the scholarly project idea being anticipated for practice implementation via development of a clinically useful "product"?
	  • Who will be the consumers of the product?
	  • What will facilitate or impede product implementation?
	  • In what form will the product be most clinically useful?
	  • Is anything missing that would prevent successful implementation of the product?

3. **The Scholarly Project Product:** Clinical Practice Critique	• What are the clinical practice strengths of the product? • What final actions are needed to allow successful implementation of the product in clinical practice? • How and when will the product be used in clinical practice? • What is the best method for presentation of the product to the intended audience(s)?
4. **Product Implementation:** Clinical Usage and Outcome Study	• How will the product usefulness or outcomes be measured? • What further improvements to the product are necessary? • What is the potential for further scholarly collaboration (i.e., further product development, research, and/or publication)?

continue their scholarly collaboration for client outcomes investigation. In this phase, scholarly partnerships will take on differing interaction from the higher educational experiences of earlier phases 1 through 3, contributing to a dynamic scholarly collaboration of professional peers that is responsive to the clinical practice environment.

AN EXAMPLE OF THE SCHOLARLY PROJECT: CONSTRAINT-INDUCED MOVEMENT THERAPY

To illustrate the MOT scholarly project process, I will present a recent scenario from the UND occupational therapy program. As a graduate advisor and occupational therapy faculty member, two of my advisees asked me to work with them in the development of their idea for a scholarly project on constraint-induced movement therapy (CIMT). CIMT is a well-researched and recognized motor strategy used by therapists in the rehabilitation of adults post-stroke who meet certain criteria (Taub et al., 1993; Taub, Crago, & Uswatte, 1998; Taub, Uswatee, & Pidikiti, 1999). CIMT uses voluntary constraint of the non-involved upper limb to promote motor and functional recovery of the involved limb over an approximate two-week period of intensive rehabilitation. Knowing that this topic had been already established as a motor intervention, we recognized that some new form of scholarship would need to take place to add to the professional body of knowledge. The students and I agreed to this caveat and began our year-long work toward this unchartered scholarship together.

After the occupational therapy student scholars initiated the discussion of the CIMT topic with me, their idea was shaped further through discussion of clinical feasibility and grounding it in the related literature. Often, the initial phases of the scholarly project involve discussion, to varying degrees, with expert practitioners in the occupational therapy profession. This collaborative discussion may take place with or without the faculty advisor present, yet is often pivotal to the shaping of the scholarly project itself. For example, how can a well-researched topic such as constraint-induced movement therapy take on a further iteration that will have meaning and purpose to present and future OT practice? During the literature review and development of the CIMT idea for this scholarly project, I suggested that the students contact regional occupational therapists who had clinical expertise in the practice of CIMT.

The scholarly project collaboration among all participants is most successful when some prior history exists between the faculty advisor and the student(s), and the faculty advisor and OT practitioners. In this example, the OT students and I knew each other's professional interests and work styles from prior coursework together. The practitioners and I had developed a previous professional relationship involving reciprocal guest speaking at the university OT classes and within the rehabilitation setting. Additionally, one OT practitioner and I had received joint institutional board approval for a retrospective research project to gather outcomes data on a CIMT outpatient protocol being used at the rehabilitation facility. The CIMT outpatient protocol used the occupational therapy process (AOTA, 2002) along with the research-based CIMT methods (Taub et al., 1993; Taub, Crago, & Uswatte, 1998; Taub, Uswatee, & Pidikiti, 1999) to provide anecdotally successful outcomes. Jointly, we saw the value of documenting the intervention effects empirically. During the research planning, we also identified the possibility for OT student involvement in the research data collection phase. The two MOT students who were my current advisees were invited into the research project on CIMT as research assistants. Therefore, the prior academic relationship between the faculty advisor and OT practitioner led to a natural invitation and participation of the students in the research data collection process, but also contributed to a collegial, collaborative relationship within the scholarly project process.

The OT students' assistance with the retrospective clinical research entailed rating of outpatient before-and-after intervention videotapes alongside the practitioner and faculty member, using the Wolf Motor Function Test (Morris, Uswatte, Crago, Cook, & Taub, 2001). Thus, the OT students meshed their interest in CIMT and beginning level clinician-researcher skills with the faculty and practitioner knowledge and skills. The OT students' knowledge and enthusiasm from the evolving learning experience led them to question how they could best encourage other OT practitioners to include this effective intervention for appropriate clients. Further, the OT students questioned how clients could best become aware of CIMT services and self-evaluate their potential to participate. These questions formed the basis for their scholarly project product or outcome.

As the students' scholarly questions evolved from a purely academic and/or research inquiry to a scholarly clinical inquiry inclusive of the evidence, the students and I met with a second OT practitioner expert to seek advice in answering their two proposed scholarly product questions:

1. How do OT professionals screen and promote appropriate use of CIMT intervention for their clients?
2. What would potential CIMT intervention participants want to know in order to self-evaluate their motivation for CIMT participation?

The practitioner expert held a discussion with the students and me, the faculty advisor, to raise awareness of clinical issues related to CIMT such as: participant selection criteria, reimbursement, traditional and non-traditional referral sources, and effective methods of client education. Prior to the practitioner expert raising these issues, the inquiry had been grounded in evidence, yet as Pollock and Rochon (2002) point out, it needed the practice perspective to infuse more clinical significance into the topic.

Following this pivotal meeting with the practitioner expert, the OT students approached the development of their scholarly project product with renewed enthusiasm and an enhanced clinical awareness. They developed two brochures: one for health care professionals to make appropriate referrals for CIMT and a second for potential recipients of CIMT intervention. The professionals' brochure targeted OT and other health care professional audiences. This brochure provided a summary of existing research and considerations for appropriate referrals for CIMT services. The consumers' brochure was written for both potential CIMT clients and their significant others to inform them regarding the benefits and the practicalities of this intervention. It was written in a "top 10" question-answer format to appeal to the targeted audience. After the scholarly project completion, both brochures were distributed by the students to the practitioners for use at the rehabilitation setting.

SUMMARY OF THE SCHOLARLY PROJECT AS COLLABORATIVE SCHOLARSHIP

The scholarly project process for attainment of a master's degree in occupational therapy, as described above, results in benefits for all collaborators. The OT students, as future practitioners, were able to participate collectively in steering and crafting a scholarly project product grounded in the literature, instilled with principles of scholarship, and guided by the clinical expertise of practitioners in the current context of practice. The OT students experienced the realities of collaborative scholarship and occupational challenges that arose at each phase of the scholarly project process. In their desire for competence in combination with the contextual demands, the students achieved success and relative mastery of their higher education experiences, producing both a tangible product for professional practice and doubtless intangible products as well (Schkade & Schultz, 1992; Schultz, 2000; Schultz & Schkade, 1992). The OT faculty advisor was able to collaborate in partnership with the students and practitioners to participate in the team relationship, experience the intangible benefits of facilitating a scholarly project toward its successful outcome, and appreciate the possibilities for future collective practice scholarship. The OT practitioners experienced similar intangible benefits with the addition of the satisfaction of seeing their practice skills and knowledge being influential to the creation of a clinically useful product. Ultimately, all collaborators were aware of the resulting scholarly project product potential–future clients receiving CIMT would benefit from having outcome evidence and practical information provided to them in an understandable brochure format.

Nontraditional scholarly projects are sometimes criticized because they lack the generation of empirical data. However, we believe the scholarly projects incorporate the evidence-based practice value ". . . that the provision of quality care will depend on our ability to make choices that have been confirmed by sound scientific data, and that our decisions are based on the best evidence currently available" (Portney & Watkins, 2000, p. 3). Master's students of occupational therapy have a unique opportunity through the scholarly project process to experience aspects of practice based upon evidence and principles of scholarship. The scholarly project process provides challenges and interaction with practice professionals that goes beyond the more traditional academic demands of higher education to promote occupation-based experiences that are grounded in the realities of clinical practice. Indeed, these experiences call for adaptive responses from the students that ring true with the realities of their future practice environments within the profession of occupational therapy.

In summary, the scholarly project promotes a natural bridge between the elements of professional communication, discovery, creativity, clinical expertise, and research evidence through the collaboration of OT students with OT faculty and practitioners. It translates Boyer's (1990) four forms of scholarship: discovery, integration, application, and teaching, into an occupational therapy context. In this scholarly project process **example**, some key elements that contributed to a successful outcome were: a prior working relationship and an open communication history; a topic of mutual interest to all collaborators; commitment toward a professional goal; a willingness to work collaboratively alongside each other; a recognition of each other's strengths; an appreciation for new learning; and an ability to take action on new discoveries in an evidence-based manner. The resulting "product" was not only a tangible tool for promoting the appropriate use of an effective intervention, but also a method for development of future collaborative scholarship within the profession of occupational therapy.

REFERENCES

American Occupational Therapy Association. (2002). Occupational therapy practice framework: Domain and process. *American Journal of Occupational Therapy, 56* (6), 609-639.

American Occupational Therapy Association. (2003). Scholarship and occupational therapy (2003 Concept paper). *American Journal of Occupational Therapy, 57* (6), 641-643.

Bowman, J., & Llewellyn, G. (2002). Clinical outcomes research from the occupational therapist's perspective. *Occupational Therapy International, 9* (2), 145-166.

Boyer, E. L. (1990). Scholarship reconsidered: Priorities of the professorate. San Francisco, CA: Jossey-Bass.

Colborn, A. P. (1993). Combining practice and research. *American Journal of Occupational Therapy, 47* (8), 693-703.

Department of Occupational Therapy. (2002). *Student Manual.* Grand Forks, ND: University of North Dakota.

Glassick, C. E., Huber, M. T., & Maeroff, G. I. (1997). Scholarship assessed: Evaluation of the professorate. San Francisco, CA: Jossey-Bass.

Hague, S., & Snyder, J. R. (1991). Collaborative research: Benefits and guidelines. *Journal of Allied Health, 20* (1), 69-73.

Hammel, J., Finlayson, M., Kielhofner, G., Helfrich, C. A., & Peterson, E. (2001). Educating scholars of practice: An approach to preparing tomorrow's researchers. *Occupational Therapy in Health Care, 15* (1/2), 157-176.

Jenkins, S., Price, C. J., & Straker, L. (1998). The researching therapist: A practical guide to planning, performing and communicating research. New York: Churchill Livingstone.

Morris, D. M., Uswatte, G., Crago, J. E., Cook, E. W. III, & Taub, E. (2001). The reliability of the Wolf motor function test for assessing upper extremity function after stroke. *Archives of Physical Medicine & Rehabilitation, 82,* 750-755.

Mostrom, E., Capehart, G., Epstein, N., Woods-Reynolds, J., & Triezenberg, H. (1999). A multitrack inquiry model for physical therapist professional education. *Journal of Physical Therapy Education, 13* (2), 17-25.

Pollock, N., & Rochon, S. (2002). Becoming an evidence-based practitioner. In M. Law (Ed.), *Evidence-based rehabilitation: A guide to practice* (pp. 31-46). Thorofare, NJ: Slack Incorporated.

Portney, L. G., & Watkins, M. P. (2000). Foundations of clinical research: Applications to practice (2nd ed.). Upper Saddle River, NJ: Prentice Hall, Inc.

Rebovich, E. J., Wodarski, L. A., Hurley, R. S., Rasor-Greenhalgh, S., & Stombaugh, I. (1994). A university-community model for the integration of nutrition research, practice, and education. *Journal of the American Dietetic Association, 94* (2), 179-182.

Schkade, J. K., & Schultz, S. (1992). Occupational adaptation: Toward a holistic approach for contemporary practice, part I. *American Journal of Occupational Therapy, 46,* 829-837.

Shultz, S. (2000). Overview of theoretical models: Occupational adaptation. In P. A. Crist, C. B. Royeen, & J. A. Schkade (Eds.), *Infusing occupation into practice, second edition* (pp. 6-8). Bethesda, MD: The American Occupational Therapy Association, Inc.

Schultz, S., & Schkade, J. K. (1992). Occupational adaptation: Toward a holistic approach for contemporary practice, part II. *American Journal of Occupational Therapy, 46,* 917-925.

Selker, L. G. (1994). Clinical research in allied health. *Journal of Allied Health, 23* (4), 201-228.

Seymour, B., Kinn, S., & Sutherland, N. (2003). Valuing both critical and creative thinking in clinical practice: Narrowing the research-practice gap? *Journal of Advanced Nursing, 42* (3), 288-296.

Taub, E., Crago, J. E., & Uswatte, G. (1998). Constraint-induced movement therapy: A new approach to treatment in physical rehabilitation. *Rehabilitation Psychology, 43* (2), 152-170.

Taub, E., Miller, N. E., Novack, T. A., Cook, E. W., Fleming, W. C., Nepomuceno, C. S., Connell, J. S., & Crago, J. E. (1993). Technique to improve chronic motor deficit after stroke. *Archives of Physical Medicine & Rehabilitation, 74,* 347-354.

Taub, E., Uswatte, G., & Pidikiti, R. (1999). Constraint-induced movement therapy: A new family of techniques with broad application to physical rehabilitation–a clinical review. *Journal of Rehabilitation Research and Development, 36* (3), 237-251.

Williams, R., Bornor, J., & Law, M. (1989). Joint university-hospital appointments in physical therapy and occupational therapy schools in Canada. *Physiotherapy Canada, 41* (1), 6-14.

New Doors:
A Community Program Development Model

Kathleen Swenson Miller, PhD, OTR/L
Caryn Johnson, MS, OTR/L, FAOTA

SUMMARY. The need to provide occupational therapy services across a continuum of care has stimulated interest in moving into community-based arenas of practice. Limited job opportunities and lack of awareness of the benefits of occupational therapy are common barriers to this movement. This case study illustrates the "New Doors Model" and describes how a partnership between the university, master clinicians, students, and community agencies can result in (1) expanding occupational therapy services to facilities that have not historically interacted with occupational therapy, (2) training occupational therapists and occupational therapy students, and (3) promoting employment of occupational thera-

Kathleen Swenson Miller is Assistant Professor and Director of Combined BS/MSOT Program, and Caryn Johnson is Instructor and Fieldwork Coordinator, both at the Department of Occupational Therapy, Jefferson College of Health Professions, Thomas Jefferson University, Philadelphia, PA.

Address correspondence to: Kathleen Swenson Miller, Department of Occupational Therapy. Thomas Jefferson University, 130 South 9th Street, Suite 810, Philadelphia, PA 19107 (E-mail: kathleen.swenson-miller@mail.tju.edu).

The authors are indebted to Thomas Jefferson University Occupational Therapy faculty, and the many Philadelphia occupational therapy master clinicians and occupational therapy student partners who have worked with us to develop and apply the New Doors Model in multiple practice settings.

[Haworth co-indexing entry note]: "New Doors: A Community Program Development Model." Swenson Miller, Kathleen, and Caryn Johnson. Co-published simultaneously in *Occupational Therapy in Health Care* (The Haworth Press, Inc.) Vol. 19, No. 1/2, 2005, pp. 135-143; and: *The Scholarship of Practice: Academic-Practice Collaborations for Promoting Occupational Therapy* (ed: Patricia Crist, and Gary Kielhofner) The Haworth Press, Inc.. 2005, pp. 135-143. Single or multiple copies of this article are available for a fee from The Haworth Document Delivery Service [1-800-HAWORTH. 9:00 a.m. - 5:00 p.m. (EST). E-mail address: docdelivery@haworthpress.com].

doi:10.1300/J003v19n01_10

pists by community organizations, and (4) a scholarship of practice that studies and supports the development of occupation based practice in community settings. The New Doors Model begins with exposing new sites to occupational therapy through level I fieldwork, progressing to level II fieldwork, and ending with creation of permanent occupational therapy positions *[Article copies available for a fee from The Haworth Document Delivery Service: 1-800-HAWORTH. E-mail address: <docdelivery@ haworthpress.com> Website: <http://www.HaworthPress.com> © 2005 by The Haworth Press, Inc. All rights reserved.]*

KEYWORDS. Academic-clinical partnerships, community program development, occupational therapy

How can occupational therapists bridge the theoretical vision of practice into reality so that people have access to occupation-driven services throughout the continuum of care? How can occupational therapy practitioners and students engage in the scholarship of practice in these emerging areas of practice? How can occupational therapists assure that people have access to occupational therapy services not only at the acute stage of a health condition but also within community programs where people learn to adapt and cope with chronic health conditions? Occupational therapists increasingly voice a need to work with individuals in their natural environments.

The "New Doors Model," which creates demand and opportunities for community occupational therapy positions will be described. This model has been successful in opening the door to funded occupational therapy positions in a multitude of diverse settings that had no previous experience with occupational therapy. The New Doors Model serves multiple functions of providing: (1) occupation-based services to community programs that have not historically interacted with occupational therapy; (2) an academic-clinical partnership, involving faculty, practitioners, and students; (3) the transition for occupational therapists to become employees of community organizations; and (4) enable opportunities for scholarship of practice to study and support development of occupational therapy services in the community.

LITERATURE REVIEW

Continuum of Care. A continuum of care can be defined as a seamless system of services. Conceptualization of a continuum of care utilizes a holistic approach to individuals who require ongoing, comprehensive services. The array and intensity of services change over time, depending upon changing issues. The focus is not on pathology, but on health and function. Evashwick (1996) conceptualized a continuum of care that includes settings such as: ambulatory care or primary care; acute care; extended care such as nursing home care; home care; outreach, including screening services and transportation; health promotion; and housing. Schools, day care programs, community centers that provide leisure activities, and work places need to also be considered within the continuum of care, although Evashwick did not include these in her conceptual framework. Housing programs, health promotion programs, community centers that provide services to individuals with chronic conditions and outreach are arenas of potential practice that have been targeted in the New Doors community program initiatives.

Consistent with Healthy People 2010 goals is a need for more practice to shift into the communities where people work, play and manage their personal affairs (Healthy People 2010; Baum & Law, 1998; Baum & Law, 1997). Community is the natural context for enabling reconstruction of lifestyles for those with chronic health conditions. Fifty-nine percent of occupational therapy practice, according to the most recent national survey, continues to be carried out primarily in hospital-related practice settings. Twenty-eight percent of therapists work in school systems or early intervention, which can be considered community settings for children. Only seven percent of occupational therapy practice, other than in school systems or early intervention programs, is implemented in community settings (American Occupational Therapy Association, 2000). The work place of occupational therapists has not yet stretched into more diverse community settings, as Evashwich envisions in a seamless continuum of care.

THE NEW DOORS MODEL

The New Doors Model introduces occupational therapy services to community settings where occupational therapy has not previously been available. The outcome of the New Doors Model is mutually fulfilling, as it provides needed services to underserved populations, student preparation for emerging occupational therapy arenas of practice, role/employment expansion for occupational therapy practitioners, and opportunities for the scholarship of practice in the community.

This model can be distinguished from other emerging practice models used in student training. This model is unlike a service learning model, where students volunteer their services to an underserved population using an occupational therapy perspective. It is also different from a faculty preceptor model in that there is no cost to the academic program in terms of faculty time or work load. The New Doors Model is comprised of three phases: (1) Start-up; (2) Semi-permanent; and (3) Permanent.

Phase One: Start-Up

Site identification. Sites are identified through input from students, faculty, and members of the community who recognize unmet needs in the community. Students in the final phase of their educational program participate in the development of occupational therapy programming in these sites. Once a site has been identified, students present a plan to the program administrator regarding the potential benefit of occupational therapy services.

Needs assessment. In these new arenas of practice, the importance of collaborating with the organization and its clients during the needs assessment process must be underscored. Students are taught to be sensitive to the culture of the setting and understand their program's overall mission, values, rules, and agendas. Needs are usually identified through client and staff interview and observation.

Program design. Based on the results of the needs assessment, students begin the process of literature review and program design. Program goals and methods for achieving those goals, when supported by literature and research, facilitate marketing a prospective program to a program administrator. It has been important to recognize that programming for community practice may involve not only the clients themselves, but staff, families, and whole communities as well.

Program implementation. This is a high visibility period when the site actually sees occupational therapy in action. During the program development experience, students spend a significant amount of time on-site which allows students to develop relationships with the staff, administration and clients, as well as develop a thorough understanding of the population and their issues.

Community sites enjoy seeing a "product"–evidence of how occupational therapy impacted their clients, made a difference in their setting, or was different from less expensive services. Groups led by the occupational therapy students, in-services explaining the intervention, and educational materials to help staff sustain programs have been powerful tools for communicating the value of the occupational therapy program.

Program evaluation. Evaluation occurs at two levels. The occupational therapy students perform either a qualitative or quantitative evaluation of program effectiveness. In addition, the site evaluates the value of the occupational therapy program at an organizational level. Occupational therapy has proven itself a valuable service when the organization perceives that the services have resulted in improved client occupational performance, client satisfaction, staff effectiveness, or decreased caregiver workload.

Once sites have had an opportunity to experience occupational therapy services, they can determine the degree of benefit they actually gained from occupational therapy student involvement, and whether it is something they wish to continue. Sites respond to the contributions of occupational therapy in various ways. Those having had a particularly valuable experience may be interested in formalizing and funding a relationship with the university in order to develop more extensive occupational therapy programming. This leads to the "Semi-permanent" phase of the model.

Phase Two: Semi-Permanent

Having recognized the value of occupational therapy services on a limited basis, some sites have chosen to develop a relationship with the university in order to establish more comprehensive and sustained occupational therapy services. The organization then implements a contractual arrangement with the university whereby a part-time OTR and level II fieldwork students provide full time occupational therapy services. Funding from the organization, which may come from new grants that include occupational therapy services or from their operating budget, covers an OTR for a minimum of 8 hours a week at a salary level comparable to hospital-based therapists. The OTR's primary responsibility is to train and supervise the students. Level II fieldwork students are usually assigned in pairs to the setting for 12-week rotations throughout the calendar year. All FWII students are required to complete a systematic evaluation of the effectiveness of the services they provided. In some cases, the program evaluation has led to formal research inquiries by the involved university occupational therapy faculty.

Phase Three: Permanent

Many of the sites housing these Level II fieldwork experiences are part of large social service organizations with dozens of programs in this urban community. As word begins to spread through the organization about the impact of occupational therapy services within individual programs, it is not uncommon for other programs within the organization to express an interest in receiving occupational therapy services as well. At this point, the organization may decide to develop a permanent, full time occupational therapy position that can provide services to a number of programs. This final step, which creates one or more new occupational therapy positions in the community, helps to achieve the goal of role/employment expansion.

Table 1 describes the types of practice settings, phase of program development attained to date, and occupational therapy focus of program development in these settings. This table reflects seven years of implementing the New Doors Model.

TABLE 1. Practice Settings, Phase of Model Implementation and Focus of Occupational Therapy

Practice Setting	No. of Programs	Phase of Model			Examples of Focus of Occupational Therapy Intervention
		1	2	3	
Homeless shelters/ transitional housing	15	X	X	X	Parent-child play programs, stress management, employment readiness, life skills
Group home/ Community residential care facility	10	X	X	X	Home management skills, leisure skills, community mobility; sensory regulation, development of cognitive and self care skills, staff training
Adult social service agency	9	X			Medication management, environmental accessibility, health promotion
Pediatric social service agencies	8	X			Developmental screening, social skills, community building
Community mental health	8	X	X	X	Leisure and social skills development; stress and anger management
Sheltered workshops	7	X	X	X	Work readiness and job skills; computer and leisure skills
Schools systems- health promotion focus	5	X			Violence prevention, leisure skill development, handwriting skills; teenage parenting skills
Adult day care	4	X	X	X	Reminiscence groups, leisure skill development, sensory regulation
Criminal justice system	2	X			Stress and anger management, social skills
Senior center	2	X	X	X	Lifestyle redesign, community building
Assisted living	1	X	X		Community mobility, leisure skills, falls prevention

EXAMPLE: WISTER STREET PROJECT

Resources for Human Development (RHD) is a large multi-state social service agency serving individuals with mental illness and developmental disabilities. The university's relationship with RHD developed gradually. Following experience with Phase I of The New Doors Model, RHD approached the university about participating in a newly developing program. The Wister Street Project was to be a group home providing services to eighteen men and women with forensic backgrounds, dually diagnosed with mental illness and substance abuse. Individuals would be discharged to Wister Street following incarceration or institutionalization. Residents of the home would participate in programming designed to promote the development of life skills necessary for moving to less structured and less restrictive environments. An agreement was negotiated with the university whereby two full time level II students and a part time OTR (8 hours per week) would perform a needs assessment and design and implement occupational therapy programming.

The first pair of Level II students began their experience in the fall of 2000. Areas identified through the needs assessment included functional and cognitive assessment of the clients, money and household management, work and productive activities, community mobility, functional communication, safety awareness, health maintenance and leisure participation. A variety of group and individual interventions were designed and implemented. Currently, students implement occupational therapy programs, evaluate their effectiveness and then refine the programs. At the time of this writing, 30 students have participated in fieldwork at this facility.

Following years of positive experiences with occupational therapy, RHD developed the equivalent of three full time occupational therapy positions. The occupational therapists provide services to multiple RHD programs.

OUTCOMES OF THE NEW DOORS MODEL

Since implementation of the New Doors Model in 1998, valuable outcomes in relationship to the goals of the model have been identified. The initiative to train students in community-based arenas of practice has yielded over 375 students placements, exposing students to issues related to working in the natural environments of people with chronic health conditions. More than 75 programs providing services to underserved populations have benefited from occupational therapy services, including individual evaluation and intervention, group intervention, and staff training. The academic-clinical partnership has resulted in the training of eight occupational therapy practitioners along with six faculty members who have worked or currently work in some capacity in eleven newly created and funded community positions. The practitioners, faculty, and students involved with the New Doors Model have contributed a variety of scholarly activities at local, state, and national levels, including eight grants, seven research projects, eleven publications, and 85 presentations. The New Doors Model serves as the basis for developing academic/clinical partnerships for scholarly practice in community settings, the natural settings where people learn to adapt and cope with chronic health conditions, or where health promotion and prevention are the appropriate focus of intervention.

IMPLICATIONS FOR OCCUPATIONAL THERAPY PRACTICE

Implications for Practitioners as Part of an Academic-Clinical Partnership

One of the first challenges is determining potential target markets for occupational therapy services. All the community programs have a strong occupation base to the interventions. Occupational therapy's knowledge base in meaningful occupation, understanding the individual in relationship to the demands of their environment, and building self-efficacy through successful experience of carefully graded occupations have been unique contributions of occupational therapy. The role of occupational therapy has been that of collaborative consultant to each agency, a role in which many master clinicians have had to develop skill and a role in which students gain experience through their entry-level education. The practitioners have also been learning how to evaluate program effectiveness through this collaboration with the university. Many of these practice areas have traditionally been administered and served by social service professionals. Part of the work of the occupational therapist has been to understand new systems of care, new language, and negotiate at each site's pace in this community-building collaboration and negotiation process.

Another change as occupational therapists moved into the community is that our services have been typically supported by service or demonstration grants obtained by the agency, rather than traditional medical insurance funding. Developing skills and participating in the grant-writing process is essential for occupational therapists as we move practice into the community.

Implications for Education

Lysack et al.'s study (1995) addressed the educational needs of community practitioners. Understanding systems of care, developing collaborative consultation, marketing, interdisciplinary collaboration, staff education, incorporating evidence-based practice and program evaluation skills are essential for success in working in the community. Entry-level education of occupational therapists must include this content, which may mean decreasing emphasis on a medical model framework. Practicing therapists may need to pursue continuing education to develop many of these skills.

Implications for Potential Consumers

Application of the New Doors Model in many different community agencies has afforded individuals services in the communities where they live, work, and participate in leisure activities. As faculty and students identify new agencies for potential community-based development, we wonder aloud, "Why are we *just now* working in these settings where individuals practice their occupations on a daily basis?"

REFERENCES

American Occupational Therapy Association (2000). 2000 compensation survey, final report. Bethesda, Maryland: Author.

Baum, C. M. & Law, M. (1997). Occupational therapy practice: Focusing on occupational performance. *American Journal of Occupational Therapy, 51,* 277-288.

Baum, C. & Law, M. (1998). Community health: A responsibility, an opportunity and a fit for occupational therapy. *American Journal of Occupational Therapy, 52,* 7-10.

Evashwick, C. (Ed.). (1996). *The Continuum of Long-Term Care: An Integrated Systems Approach.* Albany, NY: Delmar Publishers.

Healthy People 2010 Introduction. Retrieved December 4, 2000 from the World Wide Web: *http://www.health.gov/healthypeople/document/html/uih/uih/1.htm*

Lysack, C., Stadnyk, R., Paterson, M., McLeod, K., & Krefting, L. (1995). Professional expertise of occupational therapists in community practice: Results of an Ontario survey. *Canadian Journal of Occupational Therapy, 62,* 138-147.

PARTICIPATORY ACTION AND OTHER RESEARCH METHODS APPLIED TO PRACTICE

A Participatory Action Research Approach for Identifying Health Service Needs of Hispanic Immigrants: Implications for Occupational Therapy

Yolanda Suarez-Balcazar, PhD
Louise I. Martinez, MPH
Clemencia Casas-Byots, BA

Yolanda Suarez-Balcazar is Associate Professor, Department of Occupational Therapy, University of Illinois at Chicago, 1919 West Taylor Street, MC-811, Chicago, IL 60612 (E-mail: ysuarez@uic.edu). Louise I. Martinez is research specialist, University of Illinois at Chicago, Department of Occupational Therapy. Clemencia Casas-Byots is Program Director, Shelter Inc., 1616 Arlington Heights, Arlington Heights, IL 60004.

[Haworth co-indexing entry note]: "A Participatory Action Research Approach for Identifying Health Service Needs of Hispanic Immigrants: Implications for Occupational Therapy." Suarez-Balcazar, Yolanda, Louise I. Martinez and Clemencia Casas Byots. Co-published simultaneously in *Occupational Therapy in Health Care* (The Haworth Press, Inc.) Vol. 19, No. 1/2, 2005, pp. 145-163; and: *The Scholarship of Practice: Academic-Practice Collaborations for Promoting Occupational Therapy* (ed: Patricia Crist, and Gary Kielhofner) The Haworth Press, Inc., 2005, pp. 145-163. Single or multiple copies of this article are available for a fee from The Haworth Document Delivery Service [1-800-HAWORTH, 9:00 a.m.-5:00 p.m. (EST). E-mail address: docdelivery@haworthpress.com].

Available online at http://www.haworthpress.com/web/OTHC
doi:10.1300/J003v19n01_11

SUMMARY. Recently, the field of Community Occupational Therapy has started to enter into new research areas, one being participatory research. This paper illustrates a participatory research methodology adapted by community residents and a research team to identify the service needs of an underserved Hispanic population as well as set action agendas to meet their needs. In order to plan and implement health programs, community residents participated actively in the needs assessment, action agenda development and brainstorming of solutions to address health and community needs and concerns. Concerns identified included the lack of affordable bilingual dentists and youth involvement in gangs, drugs, and alcohol. The results of the needs assessment were shared and discussed during five public forums in which 180 Hispanics from the community discussed the dimensions of the issues and alternative solutions. This process resulted in an agenda of health issues and ideas for improvement from the perspective of Hispanics. We emphasized the advantages of using participatory methodologies when developing health and community services within Hispanic communities. Additionally, the implications for advancing a Scholarship of Practice agenda for Community Occupational Therapy are discussed. *[Article copies available for a fee from The Haworth Document Delivery Service: 1-800-HAWORTH. E-mail address: <docdelivery@haworthpress.com> Website: <http://www.HaworthPress.com> © 2005 by The Haworth Press, Inc. All rights reserved.]*

KEYWORDS. Participatory action research, scholarship and practice, occupational therapy

Two years ago, I (Yolanda Suarez-Balcazar) embarked into a new professional calling by entering the field of occupational therapy. Having been trained as a community psychologist, I discovered that community psychology and community occupational therapy have much in common. Both community psychology and occupational therapy emphasize maximizing people's well-being through environmental changes. Furthermore, principles, methods and theories from the field of community psychology could contribute to the community occupational therapy field. Most recently occupational therapy is emphasizing consumer participation in research and in the decision making process about services.

Participatory research (PR) and research with minority populations is one area that community occupational therapy can develop and make contributions to enhance scholarship and practice. Participatory research and research with minority populations have had a long history in community psychology; in fact, both areas are part of the core principles of the field (Dalton, Elias, & Wandersman, 2001). Community occupational therapy on the other hand, a young profession, just recently began to apply its strategies and models to study populations of color and it is also beginning to look at the need for research using participatory strategies.

Participatory research emphasizes the inclusion of community partners and members in the earliest stages of defining research questions, setting research priorities and designing intervention strategies (Selener, 1997). One of the key premises of participatory research is that social issues originate in the community and are better understood, analyzed, and solved when the process comes from the community (Balcazar, 2001; Balcazar, Keys, Kaplan, & Suarez-Balcazar, 1998). Within this approach, partners engage in joint reflection and analysis of needs and values of the community, collaborate in the research endeavors, and use findings to support social change efforts.

A PR approach to research, which has gained recognition in the social and health sciences, not only emphasizes the active participation of consumers in the identification of the values and issues of importance to them, but the necessary action steps to improve social conditions. Boyce and Lysack (2000) assert that in the case of oppressed groups, participatory approaches to research are designed to impact social conditions and quality of life. A PR approach has been included in the occupational therapy literature, mostly in scholarship conducted with people with disabilities. Examples of PR in OT include Cockburn and Trentham (2002); Taylor, Braveman, and Hammel (2004); and Townsend, Birch, Langley, and Langile (2000) among others.

A PR approach is congruent with a Scholarship of Practice framework as it incorporates the integration of community-based practice, the needs of urban communities, and how scholarship can inform practice and practice can inform scholarship, all with the aim of addressing social problems and improving social conditions (Hammel, Finlayson, Kielhofner, Helfrich, & Peterson, 2002). Cockburn and Trentham (2002) have highlighted how through PR, occupational therapists (OTs) can integrate community occupational therapy scholarship and practice. PR can also provide strong evidence for practice (Taylor et al., 2004) and increase the likelihood that services and programs developed will sustain over time (Suarez-Balcazar & Harper, 2003). It also facilitates ownership, adoption of innovations, empowerment and improvement of social conditions (Balcazar, Keys, Kaplan, & Suarez-Balcazar, 1998; Selener, 1997). Although PR approaches have included qualitative and critical consciousness methods, there is not one set of methodological strategies under PR. The methodology used in this case study, called the Concerns Report Method, is a participatory action oriented strategy designed to identify issues, brainstorm solutions, and take action from the perspective of consumers.

The Concerns Report Methodology (CRM) was first developed in our early work with people with disabilities at the University of Kansas. It was designed as a needs assessment tool to assist consumers with disabilities in identifying their community needs, ideas and strategies for action and to facilitate action to address needs. In occupational therapy a large body of literature has been published related to needs assessment research strategies (see, e.g., Black, Grant, Lapsley, Rawson, 1994; Finlayson, 2004; Finlayson, Baker, Rodman, & Herzberg, 2002; Freeman & Thompson, 2000); however, only few studies have taken a participatory action approach. One such example was the study conducted by Finlayson et al. (2002) in which the findings of the needs assessment were used to take action to plan and improve services at a homelessness shelter, which were monitored for a short period of time. The CRM is an approach that occupational therapists could use to not only identify community and service needs of a given population but also to obtain ideas and promote action, from the part of consumers to improve services. The following example of a PR approach describes the application of the CRM to identify the service needs and ideas for action from the perspective of Latino immigrants.

The Concerns Report Method as a PAR Approach

The Concerns Report Method, based on principles of community psychology like empowerment and participation (Dalton et al., 2001), was developed in partnership with Independent Living agencies serving people with disabilities. At the time, the agency personnel were struggling to find assessment strategies that were participatory in nature and that included qualitative and quantitative methods as well as strategies for agenda setting. The Concerns Report Method (CRM) is a systematic participatory process for setting agendas for community change from the perspective of those who share a common predicament (Fawcett et al., 1988; Fawcett, White et al., 1994; Suarez-Balcazar, Balcazar, & Fawcett, 1992; Suarez-Balcazar, Balcazar, Quiros, Chavez, & Quiros, 1995; Suarez-Balcazar, 1998). The CRM goes beyond being a needs assessment methodology. It has been conceptualized as an agenda setting, capacity building, and empowering approach as participants take control of decisions that impact their lives (Balcazar et al., 2001).

The CRM also emphasizes the praxis cycle of social action. According to Prilleltensky (2001) a PR approach to research emphasizes the praxis cycle of social action, which includes the interaction between reflection, social science, and action. This praxis cycle was built upon Freire's (1970) praxis framework in which an ongoing interaction between reflection and action is achieved through a process of critical awareness within the community. The Concerns Report Method incorporates the praxis cycle in the following phases: reflection of values and issues of importance to the community; identification of community health service needs; brainstorming of ideas and solutions; planning and taking action; and monitoring and feedback (see Figure 1). In this process, members of the community take an active role in the development of a health concerns survey through focus groups and interviews with leaders and service providers. During this process, a unique concerns survey is developed and distributed. Then, the survey results are analyzed, shared and discussed with the community in public forums. At these meetings, participants discuss the dimensions of the issues and alternative solutions to address the identified health concerns.

The Concerns Report Method has been used to identify community concerns of low-income families (Suarez-Balcazar et al., 1995), Americans with physical disabilities (Suarez-Balcazar, Bradford, & Fawcett, 1988), and Latinos with disabilities (Balcazar, Keys, & Suarez-Balcazar, 2001) among other applications. Social validity and reliability of the Concerns Report Method have been established. Schriner and Fawcett (1988) found overall high ratings of helpfulness, completeness, and representativeness of a concerns survey developed by low-income families. Mathews, Petty, and Fawcett (1990) calculated a Spearman rank correlation between the responses of 405 subjects to the same survey items on a survey developed by people with disabilities at eighteen-month intervals, finding highly consistent scores ($rs = .94$, $z = 10.85$, $p < .001$).

Project Background

In a Midwestern suburb, a large medical group undertook an initiative to improve the health services provided to an underserved population in their primary service area (see Ludwig-Beymer, Blankemeier, Casas-Byots, & Suarez-Balcazar, 1996). Hispanics represent the largest ethnic group in this area, constituting more than 14% of its population

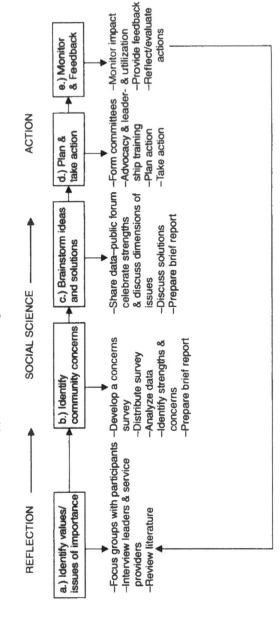

FIGURE 1. PAR Approach—Methodological Phases of the Concerns Report Method

REFLECTION   SOCIAL SCIENCE   ACTION

a.) Identify values/issues of importance

—Focus groups with participants
—Interview leaders & service providers
—Review literature

b.) Identify community concerns

—Develop a concerns survey
—Distribute survey
—Analyze data
—Identify strengths & concerns
—Prepare brief report

c.) Brainstorm ideas and solutions

—Share data–public forum celebrate strengths & discuss dimensions of issues
—Discuss solutions
—Prepare brief report

d.) Plan & take action

—Form committees
—Advocacy & leadership training
—Plan action
—Take action

e.) Monitor & Feedback

—Monitor impact & utilization
—Provide feedback
—Reflect/evaluate actions

(U.S. Census Bureau, 2000). The Hispanic population in the United States has been identified as one of the most underserved groups for health and preventive services. In comparison with Caucasians, Hispanics have limited prenatal care, higher rates of adolescent pregnancy, and until age 44 higher rates of mortality (Darroch, 2001; Frisbie, Echevarria, & Hummer, 2001). Although more Hispanics have rated their health fair or poor compared to whites, research studies have suggested that Hispanics underutilize health services and health professionals, in particular preventive services, rehabilitation services, use of allied health professionals, and screenings for life threatening diseases (Lasser, Himmelstein, Woolhandler, McCormick, & Bor, 2002; Suarez-Balcazar, 1998; Wu, Black, & Markides, 2001). Hispanics underutilize health services, in part, because of obstacles such as insufficient income to afford costly health services, difficulty with speaking English, and lack of child care, health insurance, and Spanish speaking health professionals (Freire, 2001; Flores, Abreu, Olivar, & Kastner, 1998). Furthermore, community and health services available to them are seldom based on evidence of what is important to the potential users.

In order to involve the community in the process of identifying service needs and ideas for improving services, the health care professionals formed a partnership with different stakeholders including researchers, community leaders, and residents. A PR approach (see approach in Balcazar et al., 2001) was used to identify community strengths, needs, ideas, and actions for addressing concerns.

Development of the Collaborative Partnership

An interdisciplinary and multiethnic partnership was formed, which included health professionals from a local hospital (a female physician, a public health nurse, two allied health professionals–OT and PT), a community organizer, a research intern, a Hispanic social worker, two Hispanic researchers from a local university, and three leaders of the Hispanic community. Following principles of university-community partnerships and scholarship of practice, the collaboration was based on principles of trust and mutual respect, open communication, reciprocal learning, and respect for diversity and different points of view, among others (see Braveman et al., 2001; Suarez-Balcazar, Davis et al., 2004; Suarez-Balcazar, Harper, & Lewis, 2005; Suarez-Balcazar, Muñoz, & Fisher, in press).

CRM METHODOLOGICAL PHASES

a. Reflection on Values and Service Needs

To identify community values and issues of importance, several steps were undertaken including focus groups with the community, interviews with leaders and stakeholders and a review of the literature. Three focus groups, which lasted about 90 minutes each, were conducted in Spanish with a total of 18 community members. During the focus group members reflected on issues of importance to them, their values, health related beliefs, strengths, and needs of the Hispanic community. Values such as respect, dignity, and spirituality were identified as strengths. The need for programs for adolescents and new immigrants, and access to housing, education, social support, and medical services in Spanish were identified as concerns (see Ludwig-Beymer et al., 1996).

To collect additional information for the concerns survey, we conducted several interviews with service providers from the local health center and leaders of the Hispanic community. Leaders were identified by the Hispanic social worker that lived in the community.

b. Identify Community Health Service Needs

Develop a Concerns Survey. Based on the focus groups results, the team developed a bilingual survey. Input was obtained from local health care providers, including the county health department and health care coalition, and members of the Hispanic community to ensure clarity of content and word choice. The final survey was pilot tested with eight members of the Hispanic community. The final survey had a total of 34 items encompassing issues such as dental health, programs for immigrants, housing, day care, use of cigarettes and tobacco, domestic violence, use of drugs, pediatric care and pre-natal and post-natal care, among other items. Overall, the survey included eight items related to family and culture, 13 items related to health care and prevention and 13 items related to community services for children, adolescents and the family.

The survey included two types of questions for each item. The first question asked about the importance of a particular issue. The second question asked about the respondent's satisfaction with the issue. Both questions were rated on a 5-point Likert type scale where 5 indicated not important or not satisfied and 1 indicated very important or very satisfied. For a more detailed description of methods see Ludwig-Beymer et al. (1996). One of the products of the Concerns Report Method is a prioritized list of strengths and concerns or service needs to facilitate agenda setting that can inform policies, services, and programs that can provide evidence for planning new services. Strengths are considered survey items that the majority of participants rate high in importance and high in satisfaction while concerns or service needs are survey items that the majority of participants rate high in importance and low in satisfaction on how the community is addressing the issue (Suarez-Balcazar, 1998). The process assumes that solutions to health and community problems might be more easily adopted by consumers when they are coming from community residents themselves and are not imposed on them by outsiders (Taylor et al., 2004).

Interviewers' Training and Data Collection. Members of the team trained 16 community residents in a four-hour session to ensure consistency and minimize variability of data collection. These residents received training on how to approach and screen potential respondents and on how to conduct the interviews. During the training session the mean average interobserver reliability was 97%. The interviewers were mostly Mexican (70%), and women (75% females), ranging in age from 30 to 50 years old. They were all emerging as leaders in the community by facilitating and organizing meetings. These volunteers were chosen by a Hispanic social worker that lived in the community and was familiar with the community. The interviews were conducted using door-to-door canvassing and community residents were paired with health professionals and researchers.

Survey Distribution. The sample for the survey was selected using a Cluster sampling procedure; a detailed map of the suburban city was used as the sampling frame. In this suburb, the police department was the only local department with the most up-to-date map of the city by ethnic group. The police identified areas on the map where the Hispanic population was concentrated. To verify and augment the map, 40 members of the Hispanic community marked the map with their home locations and about 100 random addresses of Hispanics (identified by last name) listed in the phone book. Every other household from each street in the Hispanic areas was selected to participate in the interview. Only one person per household was asked to participate in the survey process. The interviewer asked for the head of the household; if that person was not present, she then asked for the spouse of the head of the household. Each interview lasted approximately 45 minutes and most were conducted in Spanish.

Data Analysis. Once the surveys were collected, researchers used SPSS to enter and analyze the data. Cross tabulation of importance and satisfaction ratings for each item were calculated to examine the overall community concerns of the respondents. We also used descriptive statistics to report results.

Participants' Characteristics

A total of 210 households were interviewed. Participants included 52% female and 48% male, ranging from 16 to 81 years of age, with a mean of 35. Seventy-one percent were married. Twenty-five percent had a yearly household income of less than $15,000; 40% had an income between $15,000 and $24,999; 24% between $25,000 and $34,999; and 11% had an income of $35,000 or above. Eighty-two percent of the participants were born in Mexico. Thirty percent of the respondents did not speak English, while 37% spoke some English and one third said that they spoke English well. When asked about how they pay for their own health care, 36% of respondents had no insurance and paid on their own.

Service Needs: Strengths and Concerns. Many respondents rated several items high in importance but low in satisfaction and these items are listed in Table 1. The most common identified service needs were the lack of low cost bilingual dentists, insufficient social service programs for new immigrants, scarcity of affordable housing, lack of affordable day care, and avoidance of involvement in youth gangs and use of drugs and alcohol. Although the availability of programs for new immigrants was rated as a concern for the overall sample, it was observed that the higher the educational level of the respondent, the lesser this concern was rated as important ($rs = -.17, p = .019$).

Respondents identified a few relative strengths. Items rated by participants as high in importance and high in satisfaction were considered strengths. The most commonly identified strengths included access to friends and families to socialize and obtain support (61%), pre- and post-natal care services (61%), and utilization of pediatric care (61%). Although a high number of respondents rated pre-natal and post-natal care services high in satisfaction, it was observed that women were less satisfied than men with such services ($r = -.196, p = .007$). Differences on how both genders perceived this service are expected as women are the direct recipients of such services.

c. Brainstorming Ideas and Identifying Solutions

Share Data at Public Forums. The results of the survey were summarized in a brief report and shared at community public forums. The part-

TABLE 1. Health and Community Concerns of Hispanics: Needs and Priorities

Issues	% respondents rating item high in importance and low in satisfaction
1. Availability of low-cost dentists who speak Spanish	72%
2. Availability of programs to help new immigrants	71%
3. Availability of affordable housing	65%
4. Availability of affordable day care for pre-school children	64%
5. Avoidance of youth involvement in gangs	60%
6. Avoidance of cigarette and tobacco use	59%
7. Availability of services to prevent and treat child abuse and spousal abuse	58%
8. Availability of financial help	55%
9. Availability of services for people experiencing depression and anxiety	55%
10. Avoidance of adolescent drug and alcohol abuse	55%
11. Availability of educational programs to prevent AIDS/HIV and sexually transmitted disease	55%

Note. During the public forum participants decided to collapse issues 5 & 10 into one concern.

nership team organized four public forums in which a total of 180 community members participated. One of the forums was conducted at a local community center in which about 100 people attended. The other three were conducted in local public schools with an average attendance of 26 people. This is one of the most exciting phases of the method because during these two-hour forums, the Hispanic community was invited to celebrate the strengths, discuss the dimensions of the identified concerns, brainstorm possible solutions, and identify actions/next steps. Many compelling proposals to address identified service needs emerged in these public forums. Some of the proposed solutions included: to develop a directory of bilingual health services for Hispanic families and their children; to sponsor parenting workshops; to organize workshops for parents and adolescents on gang and drug abuse prevention; and to develop a resource list of dental services in the area. A report summarizing the data, the dimensions of the issues and the ideas suggested during the public forums was developed and presented to several stakeholders including health center staff and several service providers. This report served as a blueprint for planning new programs.

d. Action Planning and Action Taken

Develop Planning Committees. A direct result of the identification of local community needs and concerns was the establishment of several action planning committees such as one established to investigate recreational programs and activities for adolescents and another one to compile a list of health-related services which had bilingual staff. After we discussed the issues and brainstormed solutions during each of the public forums, poster paper was taped to the walls, one for each of the main concerns and participants were asked to identify an issue they wanted to work on and sign-up under that topic. As a result of this forum, community members formed working committees to take action on identified topics/strategies. Community leaders, Hispanics who participated in the development of the survey and conducted the interviews, facilitated and chaired the working committees. However, once the topics and committees were identified, participants and community residents expressed a need for advocacy and leadership training to make the committees more effective.

Advocacy and Leadership Training. Consistent with a PR approach is the building of capacity in the participants in order to enhance their ability to plan and take action (see Balcazar et al., 2001). According to Selener (1997), within a PR approach the planning and taking action steps need to come directly from the participants. In this study, the leaders and committee members were Hispanic who lived in the community. The leaders of these committees (approximately 14 people) were invited to attend four workshops designed to (a) develop leadership and problem solving skills, (b) conduct action-oriented meetings, (c) conduct action planning and advocacy as it relates to health issues, and (d) engage in critical thinking skills (see Altman, Balcazar, Fawcett, Seekins, & Young, 1994). The workshops lasted approximately three hours each and were held at a local health center over a four-month period. The leaders received copies of instructional materials in Spanish (see Balcazar, Seekins, & Fawcett, 1995) and participated in several role-play exercises to practice the skills.

Plan and Take Action. The committees used a summary of the ideas discussed at the public forum as a blue print for planning and taking action. Members met regularly to plan and implement a series of services and programs including the development of a resource directory of health services in the community with a special section on dentists and other health professionals who offer services in Spanish. Also, leaders implemented a series of educational workshops for parents, taught by

Hispanic professionals in Spanish, on how to prevent and address issues of adolescent drug abuse, as well as a series of educational and recreational activities for adolescents. Additionally, leaders developed a resource directory of facilities that offer English classes for new immigrants in the area. Lastly, the health center began providing preventive services to Hispanic immigrants.

Monitoring and Feedback. The partnership team met frequently with the leaders to monitor and provide feedback. The above actions and programs were planned and implemented with the assistance of the partnership team, including assistance in contacting professionals and obtaining resources from different service providers. In addition, most of the sessions and workshops were evaluated for participant satisfaction. Overall, most community residents were satisfied to very satisfied with the new programs and events.

IMPLICATIONS FOR COMMUNITY OCCUPATIONAL THERAPY SCHOLARSHIP AND PRACTICE

Interdisciplinary partnerships with community gatekeepers and leaders designed to identify issues and address health and service needs are critical to the advancement of occupational therapy scholarship and practice. Health care researchers have highlighted the importance of actively involving participants in the research process to impact scholarship and practice. Using a PR approach, community residents were actively involved in the formulation of the issues of concern, the identification of solutions, as well as the planning and implementation of actions that facilitated the creation of services. When problem identification and solutions are based on evidence from the perspective of potential users, ownership and sustainability is increased. The approach used in this study has implications for allied health professionals including health professionals as agents of change, as facilitators of the empowerment process of marginalized groups, and as helping to facilitate the design and implementation of community services that meet the needs of disadvantaged populations. The health professionals who participated in this research project facilitated the different phases of the PR process by serving in different roles including facilitators, coaches, trainers, health experts, and capacity builders that assisted leaders in identifying resources, as well as supporters of the empowerment process of Hispanic immigrants.

Occupational Therapists as Agents of Change. Robertson and Ramsay (1995), assert that OTs can serve as agents of change in the community-based health care system. Robertson and Ramsay (1995) have provided guidelines for developing consultation skills on program planning and development in community-based programming and evaluation sustained by evidence. Others have emphasized the need for participatory strategies within the community health care system (Rovers, 1986). Participatory methodologies like the one described in this article provide a venue for community-based occupational therapy to assist in planning and implementing practices and services that are likely to have an impact on participants' lives; this facilitates results and service utilization.

Participatory approaches like the CRM provide an opportunity for program participants to increase the input in the programs and initiatives therefore increasing the control over decisions that impact their lives, which has been defined as the process of empowerment. By having a say in those programs, participants might increase their control over resources available in the community.

OTs Meeting the Needs and Serving the Latino Population. Velde and Wittman (2001) argued that OT researchers and practitioners, as well as other health care professionals, need to develop cultural competence to work effectively with diverse populations. They assert that researchers and practitioners need certain knowledge, attitudes, and skills related to diversity and multiculturalism and need to learn about the population of interest when working with diverse communities. Given the growing Hispanic population in the United States it is important for OTs to know how to work with Hispanic individuals. For instance, OTs could assist in developing a resource directory of health services for Hispanics, assist immigrants in finding meaningful occupations, facilitate problem-solving groups on topics of importance to Hispanics such as cultural adaptation and teenagers and drugs. To accomplish this we need to not only recruit more minorities into the OT profession but train students to be culturally competent (Muñoz, 2002).

CONCLUSION

This paper illustrates a PR approach in collaboration with Hispanic immigrants in which participants formulated their service needs, and identified ideas for improvement and action strategies. The needs assessment approach yielded an agenda of service needs providing the basis for the Hispanic community to organize its efforts with the goal of problem solving and ultimately improving the quality of life and health services for their families.

In the implementation of the Concerns Report Method, residents participated in focus groups to identify topics and areas for the health survey; formed part of the research team in the development of the survey, assisted in conducting interviews, assisted in the preparation of findings for presentation at the public forums, and presented the findings to the public for discussion. The Hispanic community then formed committees to both bolster their most valued strengths and to address their greatest service needs.

It is important to highlight that four of the top service needs identified by the Hispanic community dealt with financial issues. Hadley and Hargraves (2003) found that lack of health insurance and limited financial resources were the most significant reasons given for Hispanics not visiting a health care provider within the past year. Financial deprivation is a critical issue when 25% of the respondents live in poverty and 65% receive a limited household income (between $15,000 and $35,000) with a mean of 4 people in the household for the overall sample. During the public forum, participants discussed the high cost of services (health and community) and the lack of bilingual health professionals, as dimensions of some of the problems. In addition, participants suggested that all Hispanics need to learn English and enroll in the few English classes offered in the community, in order to increase their opportunity for higher paying jobs.

The Hispanic population who participated in this study is not much different from the overall national population. Almost 36% of our respondents did not have health insurance, which is similar to the percent nationwide (35%). Similarly, 25% of the families surveyed have an annual income of $15,000 or less a year, which is similar to the statistic nationwide–about 25% of the Hispanic families in the United States live below the poverty line (U. S. Census, 2000).

As the percent of the Hispanic population increases, health professional researchers and practitioners need to know about the service needs, and more importantly, the methodologies to increase the capacities of minority groups to take an active part in decisions that affect their health and the quality of life from their own perspective. Acceptance and adoption of new programs and services is higher when participants have had an opportunity to identify their own priorities and service needs. This study provides knowledge about the Hispanic population that can be used not only to understand this group better but to design programs that are culturally appropriate and oriented toward addressing their needs.

The Concerns Report Method provides a systematic set of PAR strategies aimed at empowering disadvantaged communities by engaging in the praxis cycle of reflection, social science, and action. It is also designed to produce research evidence to impact practice by informing programs and services, which is consistent with a Scholarship of Practice framework in OT. Implementing empowerment methodologies, like the one described in this paper, increases the active role that health professionals and Hispanics themselves can play in health programming and social change.

The participatory research methodology, described in this paper, can also be easily applied to the scholarship and practice of community occupational therapy. As a relatively new field, community occupational therapy can expand to studying and addressing the needs of the Hispanic population in the United States using participatory strategies.

AUTHORS' NOTE

This project was conducted while co-author Yolanda Suarez-Balcazar was at Loyola University of Chicago, Department of Psychology. This study was conducted in collaboration with Judy Blankemeier who is a physician at Lutheran General Hospital (the institution sponsoring the project); and Patty Ludwig-Beymer, a cultural nurse at Advocate. Funding to support this research was obtained from the Chicago Land Health Initiative, Lutheran General Medical Group Clinical Research Support Grant, and the Transcultural Nursing Society. The authors thank the community members who participated in the study and assisted with this research. Appreciation is extended to Julia Trillos for her assistance in the different phases of the research project, Fabricio Balcazar who conducted the advocacy training, and Joseph Durlak for his comments on a previous draft.

REFERENCES

Altman, D. G., Balcazar, F. E., Fawcett, S. B., Seekins, T., & Young, Q. J. (1994). *Public Health Advocacy: Creating Community Change to Improve Health*. Palo Alto, CA: Stanford Center for Research in Disease Prevention in Cooperation with the Kaiser Family Foundation.

Balcazar, F., Keys, C., Kaplan, M. A., & Suarez-Balcazar, Y. (1998). Participatory action research and people with disabilities: Principles and challenges. *Canadian Journal of Rehabilitation, 12*, 105-112.

Balcazar, F., Keys, C., & Suarez-Balcazar, Y. (2001). Empowering Latinos with disabilities to address issues of independent living and disability rights: A capacity building approach. *Journal of Prevention & Intervention in the Community, 21 (2)*, 53-70.

Balcazar, F. E., Seekins, T., & Fawcett, S. B. (1995). *Liderazgo y Lucha por los derechos: Una guía práctica.* Des Plaines, IL: Genesis Center for Health and Development.

Black, D. A., Grant, C., Lapsley, H. M., & Rawson, G. K. (1994). The services and social needs of people with multiple sclerosis in New South Wales, Australia. *Journal of Rehabilitation, 60 (4)*, 60-65.

Boyce, W., & Lysack, C. (2000). Community participation: Uncovering its meaning in CBR. In M. Thomas & M. J. Thomas, *Selected readings in community based rehabilitation: CBR in transition (series 1).* Bangalore: Asia Pacific Disability Rehabilitation Journal.

Braveman, B., Helfrich, C., & Fisher, G. S. (2001). Developing and maintaining community partnerships within 'A Scholarship of Practice.' *Occupational Therapy in Health Care, 15*, 109-125.

Cafferty, P., & Engstrom, D. (2000). *Hispanics in the United States.* New Brunswick: Transaction Publishers.

Cockburn, L., & Trentham, B. (2002). Participatory action research: Integrating community occupational therapy practice and research. *Canadian Journal of Occupational Therapy, 69 (1)*, 20-30.

Dalton, J. H., Elias, M. J., & Wandersman, A. (2001). Community Psychology: Linking individuals and communities. Belmont, CA: Wadsworth/Thomson Learning.

Darroch, J. E. (2001). Adolescent pregnancy trends and demographics. *Current Women's Health Report*, 1, 102-10.

Fawcett, S. B., Suarez-Balcazar, Y., Whang-Ramos, P. L., Seekins, T., Bradford, B., & Matthews, R. M. (1988). The Concerns Report: Involving consumers in planning for rehabilitation and independent living services. *American Rehabilitation, 14*, 17-19.

Fawcett, S. B., White, G. W., Balcazar, F., Suarez-Balcazar, Y., Mathews, M. R., & Paine, A. (1994). A contextual-behavioral model of empowerment: Case studies involving people with disabilities. *American Journal of Community Psychology, 22*, 471-96.

Finlayson, M. (2004). Concerns about the future among older adults with Multiple Sclerosis. *American Journal of Occupational Therapy, 58 (1)*, 54-63.

Finlayson, M., Baker, M., Rodman, L., & Herzberg, G. (2002). The process and outcomes of a multimethod needs assessment at a homeless shelter. *American Journal of Occupational Therapy, 56 (3)*, 313-21.

Flores, G., Abreu, M., Olivar, M. A., & Kastner, B. (1998). Access barrier to health care for Hispanic children. *Archives of Pediatric and Adolescent Medicine, 152*, 119-25.

Freeman, J. A., & Thompson, A. J. (2000). Community services in multiple sclerosis: Still a matter of chance. *Journal of Neurology, Neurosurgery and Psychiatry, 69*, 728-732.

Freire, G. M. (2001). Hispanics and the politics of health care. *Journal of Health & Social Policy, 14*, 21-35.

Freire, P. (1970). *Pedagogy of the Oppressed.* New York, NY: Continuum International Publishing.

Frisbie, W. P., Echevarria, S., & Hummer, R. A. (2001). Parental care utilization among non-Hispanic Whites, African-Americans, and Mexican-Americans. *Maternal Child Health Journal, 5,* 21-33.

Hadley, J., & Hargraves, J. L. (2003). The contribution of insurance coverage and community resources to reducing racial/ethnic disparities in access to care. *Health Services Research, 38,* 809-29.

Hammel, J., Finlayson, M., Kielhofner, G., Helfrich, C., & Peterson, L. (2002). Educating scholars of practice: An approach to preparing tomorrow's researchers. *Occupational Therapy in Health Care, 15* (1/2), 157-176.

Lasser, K. E., Himmelstein, D. U., Woolhandler, S. J., McCormick, D., & Bor, D. H. (2002). Do minorities in the United States receive fewer mental health services than whites? *International Journal of Health Services, 32,* 567-78.

Ludwig-Beymer, P., Blankemeier, J., Casas-Byots, C., & Suarez-Balcazar, Y. (1996). Community assessment in a suburban Hispanic community: A description of method. *Journal of Transcultural Nursing, 8,* 19-27.

Mathews, R. M., Petty, R., & Fawcett, S. B. (1990). Rating consistency on successive statewide assessments of disability concerns. *Journal of Disability Policy Studies, 1,* 81-88.

Muñoz, J. (2002). Culturally responsive caring in occupational therapy: A grounded theory. Unpublished doctoral dissertation, University of Pittsburgh, Pittsburgh.

Prilleltensky, I. (2001). Value-based praxis in community psychology: Moving towards social justice and social action. *American Journal of Community Psychology, 29,* 747-78.

Robertson, S. C., & Ramsay, D. (1995). Principles of consultation: Occupational therapy in community programs. *Conference Abstracts and Resources,* 25-26.

Rovers, R. (1986). The merging of participatory and analytical approaches to evaluation: Implications for nurses in primary health care programs. *International Journal of Nursing Studies, 23 (3),* 211-219.

Schriner, K. F., & Fawcett, S. B. (1988). Development and validation of a community concerns report method. *Journal of Community Psychology, 16,* 306-316.

Selener, D. (1997). *Participatory Action Research and Social Change.* New York: Cornell Participatory Action Research Network.

Sotomayor, M. (Ed.). (1991). *Empowering Hispanic families: A critical issue for the 90's.* Milwaukee, WI: Family Service America.

Suarez-Balcazar, Y. (1998). Un modelo contextual de incremento de poder comunitario aplicado a una poblacion Hispana en los Estados Unidos. In A. M. Gonzalez (Ed.), *Psicologia Comunitaria: Fundamentos y Aplicaciones.* Madrid, Spain: Universidad Autonoma de Madrid.

Suarez-Balcazar, Y., Balcazar, F. E., & Fawcett, S. B. (1992). Problem identification in social intervention research. In F. Bryant, J. Edwards, R. S. Tindale, E. J. Posavac, L. Heath, E. Henderson, & Y. Suarez-Balcazar (Eds.), *Methodological issues in applied social psychology* (pp. 25-42). New York: Plenum Press.

Suarez-Balcazar, Y., Balcazar, F. E., Quiros, M., Chavez, M., & Quiros, O. (1995). A case study of international cooperation for community development and primary prevention in Costa Rica. In R. E. Hess & W. Stark (Eds.), *International ap-*

proaches to prevention in mental health and human services (pp. 3-23). New York: The Haworth Press, Inc.

Suarez-Balcazar, Y., Bradford, B., & Fawcett, S. B. (1988). Common concerns of disabled Americans: Issues and options. *Social Policy, 19,* 29-35.

Suarez-Balcazar, Y., Davis, M. I., Ferrari, J., Nyden, P., Olson, B., Alvarez, J., Molloy, P., & Toro, P. (2004). University-Community partnerships: A framework and an exemplar (105-120). In L. A. Jason, C. B. Keys, Y. Suarez-Balcazar, R. R. Taylor, & M. I. Davis, J. Durlak, & D. Isenberg (Eds.) *Participatory Community Research.* Washington, DC: American Psychological Association.

Suarez-Balcazar, Y., & Harper, G. W. (Eds.). (2003). *Empowerment and participatory evaluation of community interventions.* New York: The Haworth Press, Inc.

Suarez-Balcazar, Y., Harper, G., & Lewis, R. (2005). An Interactive Contextual Model of Community University Collaborations for Research and Action. *Health Education & Behavior,* 32(1), 84-101.

Suarez-Balcazar, Y., Muñoz, J., & Fisher, G. (in press). A model of university-community partnerships for occupational therapy scholarship and practice. In G. Kielhofner (Ed.) *Scholarship in occupational therapy: Methods of inquiry for enhancing practice.* Philadelphia: F.A. Davis Company.

Suleiman, L. (2003). Beyond cultural competence: Language access and Latino civil rights. *Child Welfare, 82,* (2), 185-200.

Taylor, R. T., Braveman, B., & Hammel, J. (2004). Developing and evaluating community-based services through participatory action research: Two case examples. *American Journal of Occupational Therapy, 58 (1),* 73-82.

Townsend, E., Birch, D. E., Langley, J., & Langile, L. (2000). Participatory research in a mental health clubhouse. *The Occupational Therapy Journal of Research,* 20 (1), 18-43.

U.S. Census Bureau (2000). *State and County QuickFacts.* Retrieved March 18, 2004, from http://quickfacts.census.gov/qfd/index.html.

U.S. Census Bureau (2002). *The Hispanic population in the United States.* Retrieved March 15, 2004, from *www.census.gov/population/www/socdemo/hispanic.html.*

Wu, Z. H., Black, S. A., & Markides, K. S. (2001). Prevalence and associated factors of cancer screening: Why are so many older Mexican American women never screened? *Prevention Medicine,* 33, 268-73.

Brief or New:
Interagency Collaboration to Support Adults
with Developmental Disabilities
in College Campus Living

John F. Rose, MA, EdL
Donna M. Heine, MA, OTR, LPC
Cristine M. Gray, OTR

SUMMARY. Interagency collaboration in provision of a campus transition living program for young adults with developmental disabilities is described. Given the current imbalance of available resources versus need for service provision, creative teamwork is imperative. Schools and community agencies interact with young adults to apply classroom learning to real-life experiences. This project demonstrates through specific student experiences successful behavioral strategies, challenges and benefits of this life skills program as the evidence of the efficacy of

John F. Rose is a Teacher of Transitional Services for the Washtenaw Intermediate School District, 1819 South Wagner Road, Ann Arbor, MI 48104 (E-mail: jrose@ wash.k12.mi.us). Donna M. Heine is Fieldwork Coordinator, Occupational Therapy Program, Eastern Michigan University, 324 Marshall Building, Ypsilanti, MI 48197 (E-mail: donna.heine@emich.edu). Cristine M. Gray is affiliated with the Washtenaw Intermediate School District, 1819 South Wagner Road, Ann Arbor, MI 48104 (E-mail: cgray@wash.k12.mi.us).

The authors thank Andrea Weid Perkey, OTR, for her contributions to this project.

[Haworth co-indexing entry note]: "Brief or New: Interagency Collaboration to Support Adults with Developmental Disabilities in College Campus Living." Rose, John F., Donna M. Heine, and Cristine M. Gray. Co-published simultaneously in *Occupational Therapy in Health Care* (The Haworth Press, Inc.) Vol. 19, No. 1/2, 2005, pp. 165-171; and: *The Scholarship of Practice: Academic-Practice Collaborations for Promoting Occupational Therapy* (ed: Patricia Crist, and Gary Kielhofner) The Haworth Press, Inc., 2005, pp. 165-171. Single or multiple copies of this article are available for a fee from The Haworth Document Delivery Service [1-800-HAWORTH, 9:00 a.m. - 5:00 p.m. (EST). E-mail address: docdelivery@haworthpress.com].

this model. The purpose of this model is three-fold: (1) to provide real-life transitional living experiences in combination with classroom learning for young adults with developmental disabilities; (2) to provide an innovative service delivery model for collaboration of community agencies utilizing alternative funding; (3) to relate the service delivery process to occupation and address the care, values, choices, needs, and interventions used to support and improve performance in occupational engagement and participation. *[Article copies available for a fee from The Haworth Document Delivery Service: 1-800-HAWORTH. E-mail address: <docdelivery@haworthpress.com> Website: <http://www.HaworthPress.com>*

KEYWORDS. Interagency cooperation, program development, collaborative teaming

BACKGROUND

The Life Skills Experience is a collaborative, transitional living program in which schools and community agencies interact with young adults (18-26 years old) with developmental disabilities, and their parents to blend classroom learning with real life.

Through this program Washtenaw Intermediate School District students live in accessible apartments with roommates on campus, learning independent living skills (ILS) as is consistent with their age group. Neidstadt and Cohn define ILS as ". . . advanced activity of daily living or community living skills that include such areas as homemaking, personal health care, and money management" (1990, p. 692). Using their natural supports of friends, family and roommates, plus students, staff and agencies, these young adults gain skills both educationally and experientially.

A consortium consisting of representatives from Eastern Michigan University (EMU), Center for Independent Living (CIL), Community Residential Corporation (CRC), Community Mental Health (CMH), Washtenaw Intermediate School District (WISD), Washtenaw Association for Community Advocacy (WACA), and concerned parents worked together to make this project viable.

Funding support was provided, in part, through the Widman Foundation ($10,000), Michigan Campus Venture Grant ($2,500), and donation of supplies and services from CIL, CRC, WISD, and EMU. The Family Independence Agency (FIA) provided support on an individual basis. Parents and students were responsible for payment of the usual expenses of utilities, phone, food, and rent (at a reduced rate through an agreement with the EMU Housing Department).

As occupational therapists, and other professionals, shift from the institutional biomedical model of practice to community practice, they must cultivate and disseminate knowledge of successful models of community practice. McColl observed, "Although we advocate community . . . without a solid knowledge base, it is difficult for therapists to make the transition to community-based models of service delivery" (1998, p. 16).

LITERATURE REVIEW

Literature supports both the need for high school students with developmental disabilities to receive more realistic transitional planning opportunities, as well as the role of occupational therapists in providing these opportunities. Here, transition refers to ". . . an all-inclusive process that focuses on improving a student's employment outcomes, housing options, and social networks, after leaving school" (National Transition Network, 1996). The importance of using natural environments in real work, educational, and residential settings is emphasized (Brollier, Shepherd, & Markley, 1994; Hall, Klienert, & Kearnes, 2000; McColl, 1998). As Davidson and Fitzgerald state, ". . . transition comes naturally to occupational therapy practitioners because our profession is based on inclusion and client-centeredness" (2001, p. 19). Recent legislation continues to support these concepts, the Olmstead Act in 1999 (2003, p. CE-5), and the New Freedom Initiative (DHHS, 2003). However, environmental supports and funding are still not readily available.

Literature advocates that adults with developmental disabilities are entitled to what Herge describes as ". . . experiencing a normal life cycle (e.g., participating in work activities, moving from family home, and beginning independent lives)" (2003, p. CE-1).

Authors support, ". . . the right and dignity of risk, the importance of community integration and the need for environments to be as minimally restrictive as possible" (Lyons, Kielhofner & Kavanaugh, 1985, p. 80). Hall, Kleinert and Kearns find ". . . the rationale to provide age-appropriate services to 18-21 year-old students in a postsecondary setting was compelling" (2000, p. 58). Further, education needs to extend beyond the classroom. As noted, ". . . a task is better appreciated in its entirety (i.e., in terms of its requirements, purpose and meaning, its relationship to people and task) when it is encountered in a natural setting" (Lyons, Kielhofner & Kavanaugh, 1985, p. 381).

METHOD

In the fall of 2001, the Life Skills Experience began. Based on a systematic approach of functional analysis, and since strengths coincide with limitations, an interview, the Canadian Occupational Performance Measure (COPM), (Law, Baptiste, Carswell, McColl, Polatjko & Pollack, 1994), and task-related assessments were initially used by the WISD OT to assess the skill level of the EMU apartment student. Results were then used to outline the adaptive behavior strategies used for working on the practical skills of daily living and community living activities. Adaptive behavior being the ". . . collection of conceptual, social, and practical skills that people have learned so they can function in their everyday lives" (AAMR, 2003, p. 3). Opportunities to work on shopping, cooking, cleaning, grooming, leisure, and safety were targeted for areas of improvement, enabling the OT to support real-life challenges. The OT's role was to help incorporate the levels of adaptations and accommodations to optimize individual functioning as part of a person-centered approach. Adaptations/accommodations were chosen for their ease and practicality of implementation for the WISD apartment student. Some examples were: using picture/word cards for grocery shopping, utilizing a planner for scheduling daily activities, providing safe kitchen equipment and picture/word cookbooks for cooking, setting up the bathroom for accessibility, and learning to use household cleaning products and electrical equipment (vacuums, microwaves, stoves, hair dryers). Additionally, an EMU recreational therapy student facilitated participation in on and off-campus leisure activities after school hours. The WISD teacher coordinated the team, WISD classroom staff members helped to reinforce skills such as laundry, lunch preparation, and community participation during the course of the school day, along with work experience.

In the fall of 2002, this model was modified in three areas. Added were collaborative supervision, use of the Assessment of Motor and Process Skills (AMPS) (Fisher, 1999) and the Occupational Self Assessment (OSA) (Baron et al., 2002), and FIA apartment support.

The WISD student tasks continued to be ". . . focused on the facilitation of learning by breaking tasks into their components and applying behavioral principles of sequencing and chaining, and cue redundancy" (Lyons, Kielhofner, & Kavanaugh, 1985, p. 381) WISD student had enough natural supports and knowledge to be functionally independent and to make decisions as independently as possible. One of the program evaluation tools was a simple questionnaire administered, using a five-point Likert scale to rate how positive (5) or negative (1) the experience was. One parent gave the Life Skills Experience a 4/5 for the experience so far and 4/5 for services received. Parents included positive comments such as "[they appreciate] . . . having my daughter . . . on her own," ". . . thought it was the right arrangement for a new apartment," "[it was good for them because] . . . both Dad and I had to let go," ". . . under the right situations [their daughter could] live independently."

The daughter, who lived in the apartment, rated the overall project a 6/5! Services she gave a 3/5. Things she enjoyed were doing dishes, her roommate, watching movies, playing cards and games, making her lunch every day, and being on campus.

The Eastern Michigan University roommate gave the overall experience a 4/5. She said it was a great experience for her as well as the student. She had respect for parents of students with developmental disabilities.

In considering the next steps, the parents would like to look for a new apartment situation if the supports are right. Both agreed they would not like to have their daughter dropped into a situation without supports.

CONCLUSION

The goal of the consortium to develop an independent living experience in a natural environment for students with developmental disabilities (18-26 years old) has been met. WISD students had the opportunity to live semi-independently for the first time in their young adult lives. An innovative service delivery model for the collaboration of community agencies utilizing alternative funding sources was established. The service delivery process related to occupation addressed the care, values, choices, needs, and participation.

There are several advantages of this project as a transitional experience. Because ". . . individuals do have genuine difficulty performing some tasks, caretakers often overcompensate by underestimating their competence and requiring unnecessarily simple routines of behavior" (Lyons, Kielhofner, & Kavanaugh, 1985, p. 378). Thus, the ". . . person may acquire habits which presume a lower level of skill than that of which they are capable," (Lyons, Kielhofner, & Kavanaugh, 1985, p. 378). Through the Life Skills Project, the EMU student was encouraged to take risks, make mistakes, and learn new skills of independence in a minimally restrictive setting. Her comment after living in her apartment for only a short time? "I LOVE IT!!"

FUTURE RECOMMENDATIONS

The Behavioral Supports policy statement of the AAMR/Arc is ". . . people with mental retardation and developmental disabilities should have access to behavioral supports that are individually designed, positive, help them learn new skills, provide alternatives to challenging behaviors, offer opportunities for choice and social integration, and allow for environmental modifications" (AAMR/Arc, 2002, p. 1). For this reason, strong collaboration and committed buy-in is necessary among community agencies and funding sources. Agency-specific roles need to be clarified and school system supports should be minimized to the hours of the school day. Networking with other professionals would help identify more resources in the community. Providing natural and agency supports during weekend and evening hours is essential. A variety of independent living and community-based skill assessments needs to be developed for individuals with moderate to severe impairments. The Learning Skills Experience demonstrates that interagency cooperation is possible. The structure of this program may serve as a model for others to build upon and to expand our professional knowledge base.

REFERENCES

AAMR (2003). Fact Sheet: Frequently Asked Questions About Mental Retardation. Washington, DC: Author. Retrieved January 6, 2004, from http://www/aamr.org/policies/faq_mental_retardation.shtml.

AAMR/Arc (2002). Position Statements. Washington, DC: Author. Retrieved January 6, 2004 from http://www.aamr.org/policies/pos_beh_sppts.shtml.

Baron, K., Kielhofner, G., Iyengar, A., Goldhammer, V., & Wolenski, J. (2002). The Occupational Therapy Self Assessment (OSA) Version 2.0. Chicago: Model of Human Occupation Clearinghouse, Department of Occupational Therapy, College of Applied Health Sciences, University of Illinois at Chicago.

Brollier, C., Shepherd, J., & Markey, K. F. (1994). Transition from school to community living. *American Journal of Occupational Therapy*, 48, 346-353.

Davidson, D. A., & Fitzgerald, L. (2001). Transition planning for students. *OT Practice*, 6 (17), 17-20.

Fisher, A. G. (1999). Assessment of motor and process skills (3rd ed.). Ft. Collins, CO: Three Star Press.

Hall, M., Klienert, H. L., & Kearns, J. F. (2000). Going to college! Postsecondary programs for students with moderate and severe disabilities. *Teaching Exceptional Children*, 32, 3, 58-65.

Herge, E. A. (2003, November). Beyond the basics to participation: Occupational therapy for adults with developmental disabilities. *OT Practice*, 8, 21, CE 1-8.

Law, M., Baptiste, S., Carswell, A., McColl, M. A., Polatjko, H., & Pollack, N. (1994). Canadian occupational performance measure (2nd ed.). Ottawa, ON: CAOT Publications ACE.

Lyons, M., Kielhofner. G., & Kavanaugh, M. (1985). Mental retardation. In G. Kielhofner (Ed.), *A model of human occupation: Theory and application.* (pp. 371-401). Baltimore: Williams & Wilkins.

McColl, M. A. (1998). What do we need to know to practice occupational therapy in the community? *American Journal of Occupational Therapy*, 52, 1, 11-18.

National Transition Network (1996, Winter). Transition planning for success in adult life (Parent Brief). Minneapolis, MN: Author.

Neistadt, M. E., & Cohn, E. S. (1990).Evaluating a Level I fieldwork model for independent living skills. *American Journal of Occupational Therapy*, 44, 692-699.

The Olmstead Act (1999). 527 U. S. 581, 119 S. Ct. 2176.

U.S. Department of Health and Human Services (2003). The new freedom initiative. Washington, DC: Author. Retrieved January 6, 2004 from http://www.hhs.gov/newfoundfreedom/init.html.

Therapists' and Clients' Perceptions of the Occupational Performance History Interview

Ashwini Apte, MS (OT), OTR
Gary Kielhofner, DrPH, OTR/L, FAOTA
Amy Paul-Ward, PhD
Brent Braveman, PhD, OTR/L, FAOTA

SUMMARY. The Occupational Performance History Interview-Second Version (OPHI-II) is a semi-structured interview that gathers life history

Ashwini Apte was a graduate student in the Department of Occupational Therapy at the University of Illinois at Chicago during the time of this study. Currently she is an Occupational Therapist with Bandra East Poly Clinic in Mumbai, India. Gary Kielhofner is Professor and Head, Wade-Meyer Chair, Department of Occupational Therapy, College of Applied Health Sciences, University of Illinois at Chicago. Amy Paul-Ward was a post-doctoral fellow in the Department of Occupational Therapy at University of Illinois at Chicago during the time of this study. Currently, she is Assistant Professor in the Department of Occupational Therapy at Florida International University. Brent Braveman is Clinical Associate Professor and Director of Professional Education in the Department of Occupational Therapy, University of Illinois at Chicago.

The authors are grateful to Veronica Llerena and Mara Levin who participated in this study and willingly explored and reflected on their practice. They would like to thank the seven clients who shared their experiences and gave input to the findings of the study. This article was based on a thesis completed by the first author as partial fulfillment of the requirements of a Master of Science degree in occupational therapy at the University of Illinois at Chicago.

[Haworth co-indexing entry note]: "Therapists' and Clients' Perceptions of the Occupational Performance History Interview." Ashwini et al. Co-published simultaneously in *Occupational Therapy in Health Care* (The Haworth Press, Inc.) Vol. 19, No. 1/2, 2005, pp. 173-192; and: *The Scholarship of Practice: Academic-Practice Collaborations for Promoting Occupational Therapy* (ed: Patricia Crist, and Gary Kielhofner) The Haworth Press, Inc., 2005, pp. 173-192. Single or multiple copies of this article are available for a fee from The Haworth Document Delivery Service [1-800-HAWORTH, 9:00 a.m. - 5:00 p.m. (EST). E-mail address: docdelivery@haworthpress.com].

information. The interview data is used to score three rating scales and complete a narrative slope. Previous research has primarily examined the validity of the scales. This qualitative study sought to understand from the perspectives of therapists and clients how they experienced the interview process and narrative slope of the OPHI-II. Clients and therapists agreed that the OPHI-II interview built rapport, generated insights into the client's life experiences, and was helpful in planning goals and services and both groups generally found the narrative slope valuable. Both therapists and clients indicated the importance of tailoring the interview process and the narrative slope to each client's unique perspective and needs. Study findings both support the usefulness of the OPHI-II and provide suggestions for how it can be used most effectively. *[Article copies available for a fee from The Haworth Document Delivery Service: 1-800-HAWORTH. E-mail address: <docdelivery@haworth press.com> Website: <http://www.HaworthPress. com> © 2005 by The Haworth Press, Inc. All rights reserved.]*

KEYWORDS. Assessment, treatment planning, client-centered practice

INTRODUCTION

The Occupational Performance History Interview-Second Version (OPHI-II) (Kielhofner, Mallinson, Crawford, Nowak, Rigby, Henry, & Walens, 1998) is a semi-structured interview that gathers historical information about a person's participation. The OPHI-II is based on concepts from the model of human occupation (Kielhofner et al., 1998). It is designed as an initial assessment to improve therapists' understandings of the life histories of clients and to guide occupational therapy intervention planning. The OPHI-II has been developed through nearly two decades of ongoing research. However, most investigations have focused on the instrument's psychometric properties. The purpose of this study was to examine the process and outcomes of the OPHI-II from the perspectives of therapists and clients. The research process was participatory (Balcazar, Keys, Kaplan, & Suarez-Balcazar, 1998; Taylor, Braveman, & Hammel, 2004). Therapist and client participants, not only provided data for the study, but also participated in its analysis. Thus, the findings reflect how the OPHI-II is experienced and used in a practice context.

ADMINISTERING THE OPHI-II

The OPHI-II involves three steps (Kielhofner et al., 1998). First, the therapist conducts a semi-structured interview that focuses on clients' activity/occupational choices, critical life events, daily routine, occupational roles, and occupational settings. Following the interview, the therapist completes three rating scales (identity, competence, and occupational settings) and identifies the life history pattern reported in the interview. The life history pattern is represented as a narrative slope that characterizes the respondents' lives by plotting their major life events on a time line. The events are located above or below a middle line according to how they were experienced as relatively good or bad (see Figure 1). The resulting plot of narrative/events shows the overall shape of the person's life over time.

PREVIOUS RESEARCH ON THE OPHI-II

The first three studies provided evidence about and sought to improve the reliability of the OPHI (Kielhofner & Henry, 1988; Kielhofner, Henry, Walens, & Rogers, 1991; Gutkowski, 1992). Two additional studies provided evidence of the concurrent and predictive validity of the OPHI (Henry, Tohen, Coster, & Tickle-Degnen, 1995; Lynch & Bridle, 1993). Two studies employed surveys to query therapists about

FIGURE 1. Narrative Slope Form

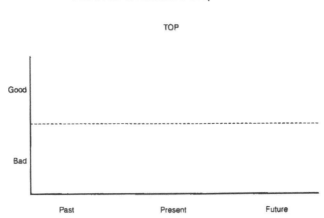

their use of the OPHI and concluded that therapists found it generally useful for clients with both physical and psychiatric disabilities and made recommendations for how to improve its administration (Bridle, Lynch, & Quesenberry, 1990; Fossey, 1996). Finally, a study by Mallinson, Mahaffey, and Kielhofner (1998) revealed that the items of the revised OPHI scale revealed three underlying constructs (competence, identity, and environmental impact rather than a single construct of occupational adaptation as originally thought).

Qualitative studies have also influenced development of the OPHI-II. For example, Kielhofner and Mallinson (1995) found that the types of questions recommended in the original OPHI and used by therapists often prevented interviewees from giving richer narrative data and, thus, recommended changes that are incorporated into the OPHI-II interview. Further, Mallinson, Kielhofner, and Mattingly (1996) found that interviewees often narrated their life histories by evoking metaphors as a way of making sense of their life situation. These findings are reflected in the OPHI-II narrative analysis.

Collectively these studies on the original OPHI contributed to shaping the current OPHI-II including the structure of the interview, its three rating scales and the narrative slope. Research on the OPHI-II indicated that the three scales are internally valid and can be applied to a wide range of persons across cultures (Kielhofner et al., 2001). The narrative slope of the OPHI-II has also been shown to predict clients' participation in and outcomes from a program of vocational services. (Kielhofner et al., 2004). To date, no research has examined how therapists use and perceive the OPHI-II. Moreover, no research has examined clients' perceptions and experiences of participating in the OPHI-II.

AIMS OF THE STUDY

The overall aim of this study is to examine the OPHI-II interview and narrative slope in use. This study sought to: (1) understand from the perspectives of therapists how they used the interview and narrative slope, and what value and limitations they saw in them, (2) examine how clients understood and experienced the interview and narrative slope and whether they found it useful for themselves, and (3) determine how closely the perceptions of the therapists matched with that of their clients, regarding the use of this tool.

CONTEXT OF THE STUDY

This investigation was carried out in the context of a larger federally-funded study "Enabling Self-Determination (ESD) for people living with AIDS" (H133G020217-3). This comparison group study is examining the outcomes of independent living and vocational services based on the Model of Human Occupation for persons living with AIDS who reside in transitional living facilities. As part of the initial assessment of all clients who are participants in the larger study, clients participate in the Occupational Performance History Interview-Second Version (OPHI-II). Three occupational therapists that are part of the study are responsible for administering the OPHI-II.

METHODS

An anthropological rapid ethnographic approach (Scrimshaw & Hurtado, 1987) provided a basis for the design of this study. This approach allows researchers to conduct qualitative data with a relatively short period of data collection (4 to 8 weeks) and focuses the research on a few specific topics (Scrimshaw & Hurtado, 1987). Bernard (1994) defines rapid ethnographic assessment simply as "going in and getting on with the job of collecting data without spending months developing rapport." This definition reflects the reality facing many applied researchers, namely limited time which precludes their ability to conduct extensive participant observation. Therefore, participant observations were conducted by the third author as part of the larger project and used to provide insights during question development. Ultimately the first author utilized qualitative interview strategies that were based upon the research team's longstanding familiarity with this research context, population, and understanding of the use of the OPHI-II in different therapeutic contexts. All of the interview data for this study were collected by the first author over a 3-month period.

Participants and Sampling

Ethical approval for this study was obtained from the University of Illinois Institutional Review Board and all participants gave informed consent for participating in the study. There were two groups of participants in this study. The first group was a convenience sample consisting of the three occupational therapists who administered the OPHI-II as part of the larger study described above. These therapists ranged in experience from one who has been a therapist for 20 years to one who was a new practitioner. The more experienced therapist, who is also an author of this paper, had done previous research using the OPHI-II and was thus very familiar with it. One therapist, with three years of experience, had previously used the OPHI-II and the new therapist used the OPHI-II for the first time as a therapist in this project.

Purposive sampling (Bernard, 1994) was used to select the second group of participants. This group consisted of clients who were enrolled in the ESD program. Specifically, there were seven client participants, (6 males and one female), six of whom identified as African American and 1 of whom identified as Latino. They ranged in age from 24 to 50 years. All the clients were HIV +, six of the participants had substance abuse histories, four of them were getting treatment for mental disorders. All were residents of the three supportive living facilities where the ESD program was implemented. Three residents were from one transitional living facility, two from a second and two from a third.

Data Collection

The data were collected through semi-structured, qualitative interviews with both therapists and clients. A separate interview guide was developed for use with each group. The interview guide used with therapists focused on each therapist's use of the OPHI-II with their clients in the ESD project, with specific emphasis on the usefulness of the narrative and narrative slope in treatment planning. The guide used with clients focused both on their understanding of the interview's purpose as well as their perceptions of the therapist's understanding of their experiences based on the depiction of the narrative slope and subsequent conversations with the therapist. The client interview guide was pilot tested with a peer mentor working on the project. All of the interviews were audiotape recorded and transcribed. Each interview ranged from 40 minutes to 75 minutes. Additionally, after a first draft of the findings was completed, brief member-check interviews were conducted with all of the therapists and five of the client participants to validate the findings (Taylor & Bogdan, 1998). These member-checks were conducted approximately three months after the initial data collection was completed.

FINDINGS

The findings are presented in two parts. In the first part we examine therapists' perceptions of the OPHI-II interview and the narrative slope.

In the second part we discuss the clients' perceptions of these two aspects of the OPHI-II. Therapists' perceptions of the interview can best be characterized in terms of their overall perceptions of the interview and their emphasis of the importance of client characteristics in shaping how they did the interview and what came out of it.

THERAPISTS' PERCEPTIONS OF THE OPHI-II

Perceptions of the Interview Process

All of the therapists viewed the OPHI-II interview as a rapport-building opportunity. As one therapist noted, "A lot of people I talked to afterwards would, when I said thank you for taking the time to do this, they would say, thanks for listening, especially since it's so open."

Therapists also saw it as an opportunity to enable the clients to think more systematically about their own lives. One therapist indicated that clients often observed that they "haven't thought about that stuff for a long time" and that the interview, therefore, stimulated their thinking. Another therapist noted, "If occupational therapy is not there in a setting, there won't be a thorough understanding of our clients, and OPHI-II interview helps us to gain this understanding. It helps the clients to open up."

Additionally therapists saw the interview as providing them important insights about the client. For example, one therapist noted, "Getting to know the person's life story is really important . . . because I think looking at that whole picture and seeing what people have gone through in the past and how people have rebounded from things in the past and how they have relapsed, in the past, can really inform you as to what seems to be really beneficial for the person."

As this therapist alluded, the information from the interview was perceived to be helpful in shaping the nature of the services provided to the clients. Another therapist indicated that the interview could be therapeutic in itself as it could get clients into thinking about aspects of their lives that they had not thought of previously.

Influence of Client Characteristics on the Interview

Therapists noted that client characteristics strongly influenced how they conducted the interview as well as the usefulness of the information they obtained. For instance, one therapist noted that how much you learn from the interview is limited by how articulate the client is and by how much the client trusted the therapist. Another therapist noted that the interview was also influenced by the extent to which the therapist shares background with the client, "During the interview I can identify more with female clients. In case of African-American clients I can't really fully identify with them, as I can with other people. I am conscious of being an outsider." One therapist noted that conducting the interview was affected by how the clients responded, "You want to make the experience safe for the person . . . where a person comes off as very open, you may press more and ask more probing questions, when a person who is guarded, you tend to not press as hard, as deeply, probe."

Therapists felt that the quality of the information obtained from the interview also was dependent on where the clients were in their lives. One therapist noted, "If the clients are in a very introspective phase, going through time where they are thinking about stuff, when they tell me their life stories they tell me events, but they also give me an analysis . . . whereas other people might just tell their story and are not at the place where they really give analysis."

Finally, therapists noted the importance of considering the interview as a flexible process to fit each client. Therapists noted that for some clients the interview was not best administered in a single session. As one therapist noted, some clients "for one reason or another don't do well with 'questions' in a long sit down interview" recommending instead that one should "gather information over days or weeks." Therapists indicated that a more complete and valuable picture of the client often emerges from such an approach to administering the interview. Therapists also noted that the OPHI-II begins a conversation that is important to continue over time. As one therapist noted, "you can't assume that your assessment is something you do just once."

PERCEPTIONS OF THE NARRATIVE SLOPE

Each therapist had a different style of presenting and discussing the narrative slope with clients. One therapist primarily validated its accuracy with clients while another not only discussed the narrative slope with each client but also gave them a copy. According to this therapist, "It's a good reminder that well I am headed in the right direction, I want to keep heading this way, what do I need to keep heading in this direction. Its acts as a good visual representation . . ."

Another therapist reported that sometimes she used the narrative slope in a group context. Clients together examined their narrative slopes, talked about them, and did some goal-setting using the slope. Variation in the use of the slope occurred not only across but also within therapists, as will be noted later.

Just as their styles of using the narrative slope varied, so did their views about it. Nonetheless, there were some common themes. In discussing the narrative slope, therapists talked about its value in providing them with insights into the client's life, the importance of calibrating the use of the narrative slope to client characteristics, its value in collaborative treatment planning, and its use as part of the intervention.

Generating Insight into the Client's Life

All of the therapists agreed that the slope was useful in enabling them to grasp a client's life. They stressed the importance of validating the slope with the client in order to make sure that they got it right. For example, as one therapist noted there are times when she is unsure of whether she has accurately understood and depicted the person's experiences. But by validating the slope with the client she has been reassured by the client's response that it was accurate and thus enabled the therapist to view the client's experiences in a new way.

The therapist went on to note that the slope can help clients, "evaluate their lives . . . having that sort of conversation with the client, what was good about this time, what was bad about this time, I think that can be very helpful."

Another therapist indicated that using the events from the slope in comparison with each other also helped to generate a better understanding, noting "I always ask things in comparison . . . Comparison makes it a lot easier for people to visualize and quantify it in a way."

Importance of Tailoring Use to the Client

As with the interview, therapists felt that use of the narrative slope had to be specifically tailored to the characteristics of the client. One therapist noted that in some instances, "Beyond clarifying the slope . . . trying to use it feels like force-fitting something. It's always a good idea to show it to the clients and verify it." This therapist noted with reference to discussing the meaning of the slope, "Not always do I want to open up that conversation. I think you have to use some judgment." This therapist used as an example a client "who had had a pretty tough go of things and wasn't a person who came in with lots of goals, lots of energy." In this case the therapist noted, "My question when I started working with her was 'how am I going to help her see possibilities?' To show someone that slope . . . would be to call attention again to . . . how bad . . . things are. If I show the slope and ask the question, 'what can you do to change this?' I think the answer is going to be nothing."

In this instance the therapist only verified the accuracy of events and did not discuss the slope to the clients because "it's just not a conversation that would have moved us forward." In the case of another client who already had goals and action plans, the therapist felt the client did not need the slope to understand his life and where it was headed. Another therapist underscored the necessity of knowing the client, in order to decide whether the narrative slope can be a useful tool for him/her. "If you know your clients then you can get a sense of who would benefit from seeing things mapped out, who would not. It has a place in therapy depending on whether the person is that kind of a thinker."

Usefulness for Collaborative Treatment Planning

As with the interview, therapists' views of the usefulness of the slope for collaborative treatment planning depended on the client. For instance, one therapist noted, "Sometimes if the person finds something new in looking at the slope, if it elicits more conversation then sometimes it can be an entry into discussing goals, but when you have not even finished the interview and the client already is able to spot out, "Here's what I want to do. Here's what I am working on, here's the help I want. [Then] drawing his attention back from that to the narrative slope doesn't get you anywhere."

This therapist also noted that when a person is not yet ready for goal setting, the narrative slope is less useful, "If the person is really in a regressive narrative slope . . . setting goals doesn't get you anywhere because you never get what you want . . . why would you pull [the narrative slope] out . . . It's not of use."

Another therapist added, "If you know your client then you can get a sense of who would benefit from seeing things mapped out, who would not. It has a place in therapy depending on whether the person is that kind of a thinker."

Use of the Narrative Slope as Part of the Therapy Process

Although it depended on the client, therapists felt that the narrative slope has the potential to be used as a therapeutic tool. In particular, they thought it could be used to give clients feedback and insight about their own lives that they could use to modify future behavior. For instance, one therapist elaborated how she used the slope to provide feedback to clients. Referring to the downward turns in the narrative slope, she noted, "Clients should be taught to identify what's the beginning of the plummet. They can be asked, What starts happening in your life when things start to go wrong? How can we kind of build some of that resiliency so that you are aware of those things trying to go wrong? What kind of supports you can use to put it back in place so that you don't have such a drop? What are the tools for recovering from something bad happening? It's heading up? Do you think it's going to stay that way? Or, Wow, this is interesting you have had a lot of ups and downs! How do you think you recovered from those bad things that happened? And asking more of those follow-up questions would probably be more useful. Can you recognize what were the factors, what symptoms, what started happening in your life that then sparked that really bad point?"

This therapist gave as example a client for whom "things went up-down-up-down, but still kind of in the middle here, then way down to her worst point, now to her best point. So it's like worst to best. And when she got to her worst point, it was really bad. She tried to commit suicide. . . . So, a therapist can stress on what was going on in her life then what were the factors, which then led to her relapse . . ."

In sum, therapists perceived the OPHI-II and narrative slope as an opportunity for rapport-building, a means of generating important insights into the client's life, and as an entrée to collaborative treatment planning. Therapists also emphasized the importance of considering a client's readiness to disclose information, reflect and plan, in deciding how the interview is administered and the narrative slope is used. Finally, therapists viewed the OPHI-II not simply as a bounded assessment, but as a process of communication that continued throughout the therapy process.

CLIENT PARTICIPANT PERSPECTIVES ON THE OPHI-II

This section first presents client participants' reactions and perceptions to the interview process and then discusses the narrative slope. The first part describes participants': (a) understanding of the interview purpose, (b) perceptions of the overall experience of the interview process, and (c) the perceived impact of participating in the interview.

Client Participant Perspectives of the Interview Process

Understanding of the Interview Purpose

When therapists administered the OPHI-II they routinely introduced clients to its purpose. This process of introducing the interview was not standardized. Instead, the therapist tailored it to each client. Six of the seven client participants indicated that they understood the purpose of the OPHI-II interview. When asked to describe that purpose, they consistently reported that they perceived the interview to be both a means of helping the therapist understanding their life experiences and present status, and a means for making plans for therapy. As one participant noted, "They interviewed me basically to set up in their program, to set up where they would know how to work with me on an individual basis, to see what I needed, take what I told them and put it with what they had, and basically see what it was what I was lacking, where I was strong at, and put together and came up with some solution."

Another participant, who reported not understanding the purpose of the interview, had a generally negative reaction to the interview as will be discussed in the next section. This participant's therapist had explained the interview's purpose but was aware of the participant's discomfort, and adapted his interview style accordingly.

The Interview Experience

Six of the seven participants described a positive reaction to responding to the therapists' questions and felt that doing so was useful. The one exception was the participant who reported not understanding the purpose of the interview, and who also felt that it asked for too much personal information, "During the interview, I gave (the therapist) some information, I didn't give him everything because I had no intention to give him everything, because I didn't feel that everything was any of his business, it was very personal, so I gave him everything that was okay."

Another participant felt that the interview was useful but expressed the following concern, "I don't think it's the greatest way to find out about a person. I think that develops over time, versus having one session to try to figure out what's going on with a person's life, I think it should be taken by steps. In my situation I would probably need more time to think about, like how I should talk about this issue, I am not ready to talk about this."

In this instance, the participant was not concerned about sharing personal information, but wanted to think about his own situation before talking it over. These findings indicate that while most clients found engaging in the OPHI-II to be a positive and useful process, not all clients are disposed to provide the information requested in a single focused interview.

Impact of the Interview Process

Participants described several perceived benefits of engaging in the interview. These included: (a) communication and trust with the therapist, (b) personal insights that emanated from the interview, and (c) influences on their own views of the future.

Communication with the therapist. Several participants felt that the interview helped them become communicative and comfortable with the therapist and increased their confidence in being able to relate and explain themselves to the therapist. Participants also reported that engaging in the interview increased their confidence, that their therapist genuinely cared about them as individuals and had empathy for their situation. For instance, one participant remarked, "The fact that she asked me and wanted to know more about it helped me know that she really cared. She was very patient." Another participant stated that "some of my experiences [the therapist] might not been through it, but of them, as a woman she could relate to my pain, . . . so yeah, I could feel that she could understand and feel what I have experienced."

Personal insights from the interview process. Most client participants reported that participating in the interview had the effect of clarifying their own thoughts and feelings. For example, a participant commented, "I could see where I am, you know, where's my strengths, where's my weakness, then you know, cause it gave time to reflect after the interview, like when I finished talking, then I could see how I feel about this, when I am all by myself, I could reflect on what I had said, and say well, I already have passed that pain, that is no longer a pain that it used to be, because, I am talking about it freely, but before I couldn't talk about it, so it helped."

Another participant commented that the interview "helped to see life more positively" and gave "positive insight about choices." Other participants' comments were that engaging in the interview "gave the ability to reflect back and compare" and "increased knowledge that we can get help when asked for."

Thinking about the future. Several client participants indicated that the interview helped them to come up with new ideas for the future. One participant expressed, "That interview made me realize that I was wasting a lot of time not doing anything, and now after the interview I am doing things that I should have been doing more aggressively, than just sitting back and waiting on it to come to me, so I woke up and started working towards those ideas."

Client Participant Perspectives on the Narrative Slope

In administering the narrative slope, each therapist took the information from the interview and plotted the major life events in the form of the narrative slope (see Figure 2 as an example).

The therapist then shared the slope with the clients in order to validate its accuracy and discuss its meaning.

None of the client participants had a negative reaction to the narrative slope. This was even true of one participant who first saw the slope

FIGURE 2. A Typical Narrative Slope

TOP

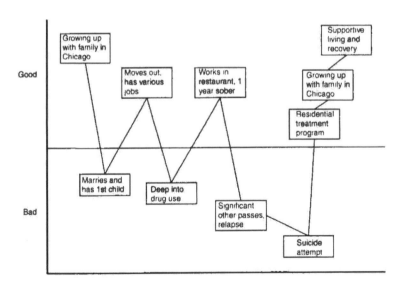

when shown it by the first author. Another participant felt that looking at the slope generated some positive feelings, but reported already having an awareness of what it signified, "For me, since I am in recovery [from substance abuse] I already know this . . . have talked about this numerous of times. So, looking at this line doesn't help cause it always with you anyways."

Another participant had mixed reactions, indicating that the narrative slope was useful because it gave him his confidence back. At the same time, he was disheartened by the realization that it was his health that was ultimately impeding his progress, "It makes me kind of skeptical about certain things, because I could see that the time I got a job or something that's where my health would come in and take the toll. Thus I can see that my health is standing in the way. That's like a stumbling block."

The remaining client participants felt that seeing the narrative slope was very helpful to them. They noted that it served as a reflection of major events in their life and helped them better understand their lives. For instance, one participant noted, "At least somebody cared to organize my life, and see where I have been, where I was, and where I think I want to go. It's helping. It was worth it, I could see a lot of things."

Several participants described the narrative slope as evoking deep feelings and felt that it was motivating for them. For instance, one participant elaborated how she reacted to seeing the negative events in her narrative slope, "No more, that's past, that's gone, what I am worried about now, is here, what I'm going to do from now on. If God gave me tomorrow what am I going to do tomorrow, not what I did yesterday, I am going to better myself."

She also described how looking at the slope gave her ideas of how to move ahead in the future. Referring to the sheet on which her narrative slope was drawn, she noted, "That's why I want to keep this paper so that I can put it in my 4th step, sometime when I feel doubt I can look at it and say, 'Wait a minute, you know that you did this. You do that again and you are going to have the same result that you had over here (points to the downs in the slope), so do it different to have a better result.'" As she noted, the line of the narrative slope would serve her both as a diary of past events and as her guideline for making future decisions. Another participant expressed a similar sentiment about the usefulness of the line delineating the slope, "Events above the line reflect what I have done and what I am better at, it's good to know."

He went on to note, "The ups in the line are motivating, because I think HIV doesn't kill me I am still alive, always look at someone in a worser situation and be grateful, keeps me positive enough to go on with my life."

Other participants agreed with his assessment that negative events below the line served as an index of what needed to be changed and that the overall upward direction of the narrative slope encouraged them. For instance, while one participant could see that his life had been like a "roller coaster," the upward direction of the end of the slope generated positive feelings and a sense of conviction to proceeding with his life. "the line going up it helps me, I am on a straight path now I don't have any crooked, no curves in my path now, don't want roller coasters now, yes, no more jumping down."

The value that many client participants attributed to the narrative slope was, reflected in the fact that they retained a copy for themselves. For example, one participant noted, "It should be given to clients, it's good to know, because the 1st thing which I would do is to hang it on my wall, then it will show me that what I am accomplishing where I am failing, where to go, in 2 years I want to go there, in 5 years . . . this [narrative slope] will help me keep focused." Another client agreed, "If given a copy that will help, it gives you a chance to see what you want to keep, what you want to throw out, what you want to change. Also . . . when I feel down, I will just look at it, because maybe when I am doing something wrong, then I might say wait a minute let me check what things I need to change."

Some clients also felt that the clients, themselves, should be given an option whether they would like to draw the slope with the therapist or on their own. As one participant noted, "I think the clients should draw the line. They have a good idea of where they are at with their life. When they see this they can get a general idea. It would be more helpful for the client that way. Therapist drawing is not so helpful, unless the client wants the therapist to help. The client should be given choice. For me it would have been good, I would include some more events."

In sum, clients generally perceive the interview as a positive experience and appreciated the opportunity to reflect with someone about their lives. One client felt the information was too personal and another preferred to have the information shared over time as trust with the therapist developed. Like therapists, clients saw the interview process as building trust. They also felt the interview gave them new insights and served as a platform for thinking about the future. Interestingly, the narrative slope had a significant impact on clients. It appeared as effective for characterizing their lives and, for several, was a potent emotional symbol.

DISCUSSION

This study examined therapists' and clients' perceptions of the OPHI-II. First of all, we want to note important limitations of the study. One limitation was that this study only focused on the interview process and the narrative slope. It did not examine therapists' or clients' perceptions of the three rating scales. Another limitation of this study was the small sample size (7 client participants and 3 occupational therapists) and the fact that all client participants were of same primary diagnoses, and were studied in the same type of context. In the future it would be useful to ask the same questions about the OPHI-II for clients with a variety of disabilities and in different contexts.

Overall, the study showed some commonalities in clients' and therapists' perceptions; both groups agreed that the OPHI-II was a good rapport-building opportunity, that it provided both the client and therapist opportunity to generate a better understanding of the client's life experiences and that it was helpful in planning goals and services.

Both therapists and clients noted the importance of doing the OPHI-II in ways that corresponded to client needs and desires. From the feedback of clients and therapists it is clear that the interview can be too much to talk about and recollect in a single session. This finding bears emphasis since there is a tendency to equate a formal or standardized interview with a more rigid administration procedure. The content gathered through the OPHI interview is standardized. However, the procedure for conducting the interview is designed to be maximally flexible. The OPHI-II manual underscores this point, noting that the best way to conduct the interview is to make it a natural conversation or series of conversations (Kielhofner et al., 1998).

Both clients and therapists agreed that the narrative slope was valuable, although more so for some clients than others. Clients who benefited least were those who had already examined their lives and were moving forward. Nonetheless, both groups agreed that for most clients the slope generated positive feelings in the clients, and motivated several clients to move forward in their lives. Both therapists and clients saw value in giving a copy of the slope to the client.

Based on the study findings the following recommendations for use of the OPHI-II can be made:

1. The interview should be used with careful reference to unique client characteristics. Such factors as the depth of the interview and whether it is done all at once or over time, all need to be fine-tuned

to the client. What is more important than gathering all the information at once is that clients are helped to reflect on their lives in the ways for which they are ready.

2. The interview should be seen as an ongoing conversation that continues beyond the initial administration. The interview is designed to help both therapist and client gain an understanding of the client's life. This understanding is unlikely to emerge completely from a single discussion. The interview is best used as a key event to begin a process in which the client's life serves as the central consideration for setting ongoing therapy goals and strategies.

3. Validation of the narrative slope with the client is always important. Since clients appear to have a strong reaction to the slope, the therapist should involve the client as much as possible in the construction of the slope. While the original OPHI-II procedure was that the therapist would create the slope after the interview and then validate it with the client, it appears that, for many clients, the narrative slope is best completed as part of the interview process. Therefore, when judged capable and motivated, clients should be invited to participate in drawing their narrative slopes along with the therapist. Finally, clients should be offered a copy of their own narrative slope.

In sum, this study examined the process of using the OPHI-II from clients' and therapists' perspectives. While the development and validation of standardized assessments is essential for evidence-based practice, it is also important to investigate how assessments play out in actual use. Further examination of this and other standardized assessments could contribute to a better understanding of how to optimize their use in everyday practice.

REFERENCES

Balcazar, F. E., Keys, C. B., Kaplan, D. L., & Suarez-Balcazar, Y. (1998). Participatory action research and people with disabilities: Principles and challenges. *Canadian Journal of Rehabilitation, 12*, 105-112.

Bernard, H. R. (1994). *Research Methods in Anthropology: Qualitative and Quantitative Approaches* (3rd ed.). CA: Sage.

Bridle, M. J., Lynch, K. B., & Quesenberry, C. M. (1990). Long term function following the central cord syndrome. *Paraplegia, 28*, 178-185.

Fossey, E. (1996). Using the Occupational Performance History Interview (OPHI): Therapists' reflections. *British Journal of Occupational Therapy, 59 (5)*, 223-228.

Gutkowski, L. E. (1992). *A generalizability study of the revised Occupational Performance History Interview.* Unpublished master's thesis, University of Illinois at Chicago.

Helfrich, C. A., & Kielhofner, G. (1994). Volitional narratives and the meaning of therapy. *American Journal of Occupational Therapy, 48,* 318-326.

Helfrich, C. A., Kielhofner, G., & Mattingly, C. (1994). Volition as narrative: An understanding of motivation in chronic illness. *The American Journal of Occupational Therapy, 42,* 311-317.

Henry, A. D., Tohen, M., Coster, W. J., & Tickle-Degnen, L. (1995). Predicting psychosocial functioning and symptomatic recovery of young adolescents and young adults following a first psychotic episode. Boston, MA (Unpublished paper).

Kielhofner, G. (2002). *A Model of Human Occupation: Theory and Application (3rd ed.).* Philadelphia: Lippincott Williams & Wilkins.

Kielhofner, G., & Henry, A. D. (1988). Development and investigation of the Occupational Performance History Interview. *American Journal of Occupational Therapy, 42,* 489-498.

Kielhofner, G., Henry, A. D., Walens, D., & Rogers, E. S. (1991). A generalizability study of the Occupational Performance History Interview. *Occupational Therapy Journal of Research, 11,* 292-306.

Kielhofner, G., & Mallinson, T. (1995). Gathering narrative data through interviews: Empirical observations and suggested guidelines. *Scandinavian Journal of Occupational Therapy, 2,* 63-68.

Kielhofner, G., Mallinson, T., Crawford, C., Nowak, M., Rigby, M., Henry, A., & Walens, D. (1998). *A user's manual for the Occupational Performance History Interview OPHI-II (version 2.0)* Chicago: the Model of Human Occupation Clearinghouse, University of Illinois at Chicago.

Kielhofner, G., Mallinson, T., Forsyth, K., & Lai, J. S. (2001). Psychometric properties of the second version of the Occupational Performance History Interview (OPHI-II). *American Journal of Occupational Therapy, 55 (3),* 260-267.

Kielhofner, G., Braveman, B., Finlayson, M., Paul-Ward, A., Goldbaum, L., & Goldstein, K. (2004). Outcomes of a vocational program for persons living with AIDS. *American Journal of Occupational Therapy, 58,* 64-72.

Law, M., Polatajko, H., Baptiste, S., & Townsend, E. (1997). Core concepts of occupational therapy. In E. Townsend (Ed.), *Enabling Occupation: An occupational therapy perspective* (pp. 29-56). Ottawa, Ontario: CAOT Publications ACE.

Lynch, K., & Bridle, M. (1993). Construct validity of the Occupational Performance History Interview. *Occupational Therapy Journal of Research, 13,* 231-240.

Mallinson, T., Kielhofner, G., & Mattingly, C. (1996). Metaphor and meaning in a clinical interview. *American Journal of Occupational Therapy, 50,* 338-346.

Mallinson, T., Mahaffey, L., & Kielhofner, G. (1998). The occupational performance history interview: Evidence for three underlying constructs of occupational adaptation. *Canadian Journal of Occupational Therapy, 65 (4),* 219-228.

Scrimshaw, S. C. M., & Hurtado, E. (1987). *Rapid Assessment Procedures for Nutrition and Primary Health Care.* Los Angeles: University of California at Los Angeles, Latin American Center Publications.

Taylor, R., Braveman, B., & Hammel, J. (2004). Developing and evaluating community services through Participatory Action Research: Two case examples. *American Journal of Occupational Therapy 58*, 35-43.

Taylor, S. J., & Bogdan, R. (1998). *Introduction to qualitative research methods: A guidebook and resource* (3rd ed.). New York: John Wiley & Sons, Inc.

Wilkins, S., Pollack, N., Rochon, S., & Law, M. (2001). Implementing client-centered practice: Why is it so difficult to do? *Canadian Journal of Occupational Therapy, 68 (2)*, 70-79.

Education and Practice Collaborations: A Pilot Case Study Between a University Faculty and County Jail Practitioners

Patricia Crist, PhD, OTR/L, FAOTA
Andrea Fairman, MOT, OTR/L
Jaime Phillip Muñoz, PhD, OTR/L, FAOTA
Anne Marie Witchger Hansen, MS, OTR/L
John Sciulli, MOT, OTR/L
Mila Eggers, MOT, OTR/L

Patricia Crist is Chairperson and Professor, Andrea Fairman is Graduate Research Assistant, Jaime Phillip Muñoz is Associate Professor, Anne Marie Witchger Hansen is Instructor and Practice-Scholar Coordinator, all at Duquesne University. John Sciulli and Mila Eggers are Occupational Therapist/Reintegration Specialists for the Goodwill Industries of Pittsburgh.

The authors would like to thank Mike Olack (Director of Community Reintegration Project for Goodwill Industries) and Eric Yenerall (Assistant Vice-President of Goodwill Industries of Pittsburgh); Jack Pischke (ACJ Inmate Program Administrator) and Ron Quinn and Ruth Howze (Allegheny County Department of Health and Human Services); Dan Goldriech (Occupational Therapy at Duquesne University) and Kelly Gaguzis-Joyce) (a Practice-Scholar in the Program during year 2) for collaborating with them through this project. Each specific contribution lead to the outcomes here and forthcoming reports that will further the evidence of occupational therapy's role in the jail setting.

[Haworth co-indexing entry note]: "Education and Practice Collaborations: A Pilot Case Study Between a University Faculty and County Jail Practitioners." Crist et al. Co-published simultaneously in *Occupational Therapy in Health Care* (The Haworth Press, Inc.) Vol. 19, No. 1/2, 2005, pp. 193-210; and: *The Scholarship of Practice: Academic-Practice Collaborations for Promoting Occupational Therapy* (ed: Patricia Crist, and Gary Kielhofner) The Haworth Press, Inc., 2005, pp. 193-210. Single or multiple copies of this article are available for a fee from The Haworth Document Delivery Service [1-800-HAWORTH, 9:00 a.m. - 5:00 p.m. (EST). E-mail address: docdelivery@haworthpress.com].

Available online at http://www.haworthpress.com/web/OTHC
doi:10.1300/J003v19n01_14

SUMMARY. The purpose of this case study is to present a partnership between faculty and practitioners that initiated a systematic evaluation data collection approach to support program development and study practice in a newly developing occupational therapy program. The Department of Occupational Therapy at Duquesne University collaborated with Goodwill Industries of Pittsburgh to introduce occupational therapy as part of a grant-supported community re-integration program at the Allegheny County Jail. In developing the program, the absence of published data regarding the occupational needs among jail inmates was evident.

This paper is presented as a case study to demonstrate that faculty-practitioner collaborations can promote the implementation of a viable, systematic evaluation process when implemented as soon as possible in the practice setting. The community-university partnership ensured that a wide variety of knowledge and resource applied to the development of an evaluation process that generated relevant data for each of the partners. The intent of providing systematic evidence for practice can enhance the intervention process and provide valuable professional information.

This paper also presents pilot descriptive results from the Occupational Self Assessment (2002) from the initial 67 (61 men & 6 women) inmates in the local Allegheny County Jail Community regarding perceptions of their own occupational competence and of the impact of their environment on their overall occupational adaptation. Using OSA responses, a difference score between reported occupational competence in an activity (rated low) and the correlated importance of the occupation (rated high), the top eight occupational performance areas of concern were identified for the total group, men only and women only. Caution in using the woman data due to the small *n* is advised. The top eight occupational performance areas of concern for this population included managing my finances, handling my responsibilities, working towards my goals, accomplishing what I set out to do, a place to live and take care of myself, basic things I need to live and take care of myself, things I need to be productive, and a place where I can be productive. Notably, four of these eight items captured the inmates' perceptions of the impact of the environment on their occupational adaptation. This study demonstrates the viability of the academic-practice partnership to support the scholarship of practice and provide a model to embed evidence-gathering through systematic evaluation processes. *[Article copies available for a fee from The Haworth Document Delivery Service: 1-800-HAWORTH. E-mail address: <docdelivery@haworthpress.com> Website: <http://www.HaworthPress.com> © 2005 by The Haworth Press, Inc. All rights reserved.]*

KEYWORDS. Incarceration, jail, partnerships

INTRODUCTION

Problem/Need

Over 2 million men and women are incarcerated in the United States and the rate of incarceration in the U.S. outpaces all other industrialized nations (Department of Justice, 2003). Incarceration is not a deterrent to future criminal acts. In fact, two thirds released from our criminal systems are rearrested in three years. One third return to some type of correctional institution within 6 months of release and one half by the end of the first year (Langan & Levin, 2002). With the decrease of pre-release education and vocational program in the 1990's, the problem worsened significantly (Lynch & Sabol, 2001). The inability of incarcerated men and women to successfully return to productive, healthy lifestyles is a major social problem. Successfully reducing recidivism among individuals who have been incarcerated can enhance individual's health, quality of life and independence. Reducing re-incarceration rates can also reduce public expenditures and provide increased public safety (Calvin Lightfoot, personal communication). "This dramatic increase in incarceration rates has been a significant growth in public-sector spending." Furthermore, Greenfeld (1985) estimated that about 60% of the individuals admitted to prison in any year have been in prison before. (Needles, 1996). With incarceration currently one of the fastest growing industries in the U.S. (Benson, 1998), reversing current trends are mandated.

Recently, community re-entry services for incarcerated populations have been advocated to address this growing crisis in the United States (Pertersilia, 2000). Occupational therapists can bring a unique perspective to the development of community re-entry programs using our understanding of occupational functioning including roles, habits, self-efficacy, and time use (Dressler & Snively, 1998; Scaffa, 2001, Cara & MacRae, 2005). Overall, however, little research is available to document the occupational priorities and needs of individuals who have been incarcerated, especially in the county jail system as compared to prisons. The difference in the two populations is that typically jail inmates are convicted of lesser offenses resulting in incarceration duration of less than two years, whereas, inmates in prison have been convicted of more serious crimes and are being held for longer terms. The short term stays in jail ultimately leads to greater challenges to prevent recidivism and re-incarceration. This paper focuses on the county jail population that frequently return to faulty habits and living environments upon release after these shorter term stays.

The purpose of this case study is to present a partnership between faculty and community-based practitioners that initiated an evaluation process in a newly developing occupational therapy program at the county jail. A primary objective to be served through this partnership was to develop a 'best practices' program where evaluation data not only guided intervention planning but over time, would result in program and knowledge development contributing to occupational therapy through collaborative studies by the partnership. The partners believed that the approach of making outcomes data central to initial program development would result in accumulating usable data from program participants over time to better understand the population's needs and facilitate meaningful, evidence-based program development in occupational therapy.

This case study will demonstrate that faculty-practitioner partnership can ensure that systematic evaluation processes are implemented in the beginning of a program to serve both individual intervention planning as well as research regarding occupational therapy services efficacy and effectiveness. The result is that information can be accumulated and studied very quickly so that practitioners better understand their population and service while contributing to the knowledge base supporting occupational therapy practice. The contemporary habit of systematic evaluation processes for data analysis is important to include in the roles and functions of all practitioners. Further, partnerships with university faculty to co-design the evaluation process with the intent of providing evidence for practice can enhance the evaluation development process and provide support for practitioners to embed scholarly activities into everyday practice. Unfortunately, in practice, service provision is expected to be implemented immediately, seldom allowing time for the practitioner to consider evaluation as anything other than a measure of individual abilities or inabilities for intervention planning. The faculty-practitioner partnership provided support to include an occupational therapy-specific evaluation process from the beginning.

Research on OT in Incarceration

Wilcock (1998) has provided a conceptual framework for understanding factors that may influence an offender's occupational functioning and overall health. These factors include occupational imbalance, occupational deprivation, and occupational alienation. Each of these factors has relevance for incarcerated populations. Whiteford (2000), drawing upon results from her completion of an occupational needs assessment in a high security Australian prison, argued that occupational deprivation was a significant barrier to community reintegration and that the men had become so estranged from occupational roles of community life and the need to structure their time to meet the challenges of community participation that the likelihood of adaptive community reintegration was significantly diminished. Diminished capacities, self-efficacy and identity as a citizen of the community are all hypothesized as byproducts of occupational deprivation. However, if time in jail is occupied with tasks related to community re-integration, can the impact of occupational deprivation be lessened?

Rehabilitation of the criminal offender has been traditionally regarded with a degree of negativism. Recently some progress has been made in connecting theoretical information to empirical research in this area. Jones and McColl (1991) looked at the evaluation of program outcomes of provision of life skills groups as an OT intervention in the prison system. These researchers found that participating in the groups had a positive impact on the inmates' volition. Specifically, these interventions improved the prisoners' "self-perceived ability to learn and perform pro-social group roles" (Jones & McColl, 1991, p. 88). The context for jails is different than prisons, meaning that the design, implementation as well as results of community re-integration programming may be different.

Case Study

An innovative, community partnership was begun in 2001 between Goodwill Industries of Pittsburgh and the Department of Occupational Therapy at Duquesne University at the Allegheny County Jail in Pittsburgh Pennsylvania to develop community re-entry programs focused on community living and vocational skills for inmates who were within 6 months of release. The project was to engage jail inmates in skill development to support community re-integration and employment for one year following release to establish more healthy behaviors that prevent recidivism and increase productive life.

One of the major strengths cited by the funding source was the partnership between University faculty resources and Goodwill's mature community programs. This program for the Allegheny County Jail opened the door for the first time to provide occupational therapy services in this setting. The project was funded primarily through various grant funds awarded though the Allegheny County Department of Health and Human Services who actively supported the initiative in the jail. Innovative educational services and interventions were commenced prior to release in order to: (1) change habit patterns; (2) consider work behaviors and employment options; and (3) develop inmate-practitioner relationships pre-release in order to sustain post-release support for engagement in a new, productive lifestyle upon release. Thus, the role of the occupational therapists became central to the community re-entry process. The specific details of this Allegheny County Jail Community Re-entry Project are discussed in earlier publications (Eggers, Scuilli, Gauguzis, & Muñoz, 2003; Eggers, Muñoz, Scuilli, & Crist, in review). Initially, the project was primarily focused on post-release employment. The collaborators quickly recognized the necessity of developing the community life skills and habits that supported the maintenance of post-release employment.

The University's goal for the Goodwill partnership was to develop a 'best practices' model to be used in other jails for teaching and scholarship purposes. Our practitioners at the jail were clinical faculty hired by the grant with the assistance of Duquesne University academic faculty. The academic faculty was particularly interested in hiring practitioners who could seamlessly engage in practice-relevant scholarship as part of everyday service delivery.

The project team hypothesized that to increase successful maintenance of a healthy lifestyle and employability and to decrease recidivism or possibly a return to criminal behaviors, the program would need to emphasize community living skill development, supportive post release relationships with a project staff, and the establishment of clear and consistent lifestyle and employment goals.

Occupational therapy's role or intervention was to design and implement a community living skills program focusing on inmate needs to decrease recidivism. With a paucity of literature on the documented occupational needs of this population, the program was initiated by drawing from the general literature. The faculty and practitioners engaged in this project knew that they needed more information about the specific occupational needs and goals of jail inmates regarding community living skills. Coupled with the knowledge that no literature existed relevant for this population and problem, the partnership saw an opportunity to develop an evaluation program that would provide information specific to the occupational needs of each inmate in the project for intervention planning but, that over time, the data could be compiled to describe the occupational needs of this population for program development and research purposes, ultimately contributing to the evidence in occupational therapy.

Notification to staff of an inmate's release from jail can be announced suddenly by the court system and for over 70% of the population, this resulted in recidivism within one year. While the overall project is showing less than 20% recidivism rate among inmates seen within our intense community re-integration program, little is known about the contribution regarding OT to this significant change (Eggers et al., in review). The Goodwill project director reported that the key difference in on-going jail programs and this partnership is the presence of occupational therapists. In partnership with university faculty, the occupational therapy staff has created an approach to reducing recidivism that is grounded in an occupational perspective emphasizing lifestyle redevelopment that integrates life skills with new patterns of habits and roles that support successful community reintegration.

From the beginning of the grant-funded project, a group of University faculty vested in the project and practitioners hired as University clinical faculty through grant dollars, met to discuss program strategies and to develop researchable ideas every 2-3 weeks. The project partners shared several common objectives; to identify the specific community re-entry needs from the inmates themselves in order to individualize interventions, to develop educational programs that would support post-release success, and to demonstrate changes resulting from the occupational therapy program. The University faculty brought to the partnership extensive knowledge and resources regarding evaluation, evidence-based practice and scholarly approaches. The clinical faculty, called Practice-Scholars, were practitioners stating interest in modeling a new approach and role to practice which embedded the scholarship of practice in everyday service delivery. The practitioners were given the title of Practice-Scholars to reflect the engagement in the scholarship of practice to support the goals for this project.

The initial meetings with faculty and the practice-scholars, centered on development of the practitioners as practice-scholars as all were new to the jail context; needed support with program development to demonstrate 'best practices' and were acquiring skills related to evidenced-based programming. These meetings were also a time of reflection on unexpected challenges where faculty and the practice scholars could brainstorm resolutions of problems. The lead Practice-Scholar on this project came from several years of practice in physical rehabilitation. The second position, and for year two, the third position were occupied by new entry-level occupational therapy practitioners. While advanced practitioners were desired in these roles, all were new to the context and this type of setting. As a result, faculty took the lead through these initial meetings to develop beneficial practice-scholar skills sets. One of these was skills sets was to develop a systematic evaluation process to be implemented and overseen by the lead practice-scholar at the jail that would result in data for analysis for occupational therapy program development and outcomes as well as individual intervention planning. The evaluation process was designed to be embedded seamlessly in daily practices and to be meaningfully-related to the overall goals of the project. Thus, the Practice-Scholars, after reviewing numbers of potential instruments for utility and quality including consultation with faculty, chose the OSA as the first assessment to be uniformly administered to inmates seen in this project. The evaluation process was structured such that the OSA could be re-administered later to measure progress and/or self-perceived changes in occupational competence between initial and discharge sessions.

The pilot results presented here will be a descriptive analysis of the occupational needs and interests of the first inmates seen in this program during the initial evaluation session. Due to program capacity and that it takes over a year to progress through the entire community re-integration program, only initial OSA data is reported here. This pilot data provides not only evidence of the success of faculty-practitioner partnerships but also, collaborative initial insight into the first published data regarding the reported occupational competence of inmates which can begin to guide practice within jail settings. This study is an attempt to begin to understand the potential role and efficacy of occupational therapy services with adults incarcerated in a county jail.

METHODS

This is a pilot study of the self-reported perception of inmates incarcerated in a county jail regarding their occupational adaptation who were currently incarcerated in a county jail and being evaluated for admission to a new program focusing on employment and community re-integration. This study only includes the initial occupational therapy evaluation for each inmate that occurred over the first 36 months of the grant. The follow-up assessment data is not analyzed here as the total number is not yet sufficient.

Subjects

Subjects included 67 inmates incarcerated at the Allegheny County Jail (ACJ) in Pittsburgh, Pennsylvania. To be included in the project, inmates had to be serving sentences with no outstanding detainers or warrants and have a projected release from the jail no more than 190 days away. These stipulations are necessary to ensure that these offenders have full opportunity to participate in the program. All participants completed the initial evaluation phase in occupational therapy. Table 1 summarizes the demographic variables for the total group (n = 67) plus separately for women (n = 6) and men (n = 61). These variables were selected from many collected as part of this project as they relate best to understanding current factors influencing inmates at the time of initial evaluation.

All data for women is to be considered with caution as the size of the group is very small but also reflects the gender proportions typically housed within the jail. The sample in this study is preponderantly male, age 33, and Black/African American with an average of 4.5 previous incarcerations. This last fact substantiates the critical need for rehabilitation programs like this to lower recidivism in the jail population. Also, over 85% use/abuse drugs which is reason the project has substance abuse counseling included.

Instruments

The Occupational Self Assessment (Version 1.0) (Baron, Keilhofner, Goldhammer, & Wolenski, 1999)

The Occupational Self Assessment (OSA) is an evaluation tool and outcome measure based on the Model of Human Occupation (MOHO) (Kielhofner, 1995). The OSA is designed as a client-centered self-report assessment that elicits an individual's perception of their own occupational competence and of the impact of their environment on their occupational adaptation. The primary factors influencing an individual's occupational behaviors include: (1) volition–referring to the process by which a person experiences, interprets, anticipates and chooses occupational behaviors; (2) habituation–referring to the maintenance of patterns of behavior in everyday life; (3) performance–referring to innate capacities, that serve as the foundation for skilled abilities; and (4) social and physical environment–includes space and objects as well as types of occupations and other persons. These factors interact to in-

TABLE 1. Demographics on Inmates

		Total Group: N = 67		Male: N = 61		Female: N = 6	
Inmates' Age (at time of assessment)	mean =	33.4		33.6		31.8	
	range =	18 - 68 yrs.		20 - 68 yrs.		28 - 36 yrs.	
	s.d.=	10.4		10.8		2.6	
Ethnicity (categories) Black/African American, White/Caucasian, Asian/Pacific Islander, Native American, Hispanic & Other	Black /African American	48		44		4	
	White/Caucasian	15		13		2	
	Native American	1		1		0	
	No reply	1		1		0	
Number of times incarcerated	mean =	4.5		4.6		3.8	
	range =	1 - 20		1 - 20		3 - 6	
	s.d.=	3.5		3.6		1.2	
		Number	%	Number	%	Number	%
Reason for incarceration Most frequent reasons listed "Other" Includes: RSP, Terrorist Threats, Public Intoxication, Civil contempt, Aggravated Assault, Firearms w/o license, unauthorized use of auto/vehicle, trespassing, Theft by Deception, 2nd offense & Robbery	Probation Violation	11	16.4%	9	14.8%	2	33.3%
	Child-custody/ support	7	10.4%	7	11.5%	0	0
	PWID	7	10.4%	7	11.5%	0	0
	Possession of Drugs	7	10.4%	7	11.5%	0	0
	Retail Theft	4	6%	3	4.9%	1	16.7%
	Burglary	3	4.5%	3	4.9%	0	0
	Simple Assault	3	4.5%	3	4.9%	0	0
	Other (see left)	18	27.9%	15	24.6%	3	50%
	DNR (did not respond)	7	10.4%	7	11.5%	0	0
Living situation prior to Incarceration	Live w/family	32	47.8%	31	50.8%	1	16.7%
	Live w/friend(s)	12	17.9%	9	14.8%	3	50%
	Rent	8	11.9%	8	13.1%	0	0%
	Homeless	8	11.9%	8	13.1%	0	0%
	Own	3	4.5%	2	3.3%	1	16.7%
	DNR	4	6%	3	4.9%	1	16.7%
Does Respondent have children?	YES -	46	68.7%	41	67.2%	5	83.3%
	NO -	21	31.3%	20	32.8%	1	16.7%
Employment status prior to incarceration	Employed -	43	64.2%	40	65.6%	3	50%
	Unemployed -	21	31.3%	18	29.5%	3	50%
	DNR -	3	4.5%	3	4.9%	0	0
Highest level of education attained- (% responded)		-YES-	-NO-	-YES-	-NO-	-YES-	-NO-
High School Diploma -		44.8%	53.7%	45.9%	52.5%	33.3%	66.7%
Earned GED		35.8%	28.4%	41.2%	35.3%	50%	16.7%
Technical School		26.9%	67.2%	29.5%	63.9%	0 %	100%
Some Credits/College Grad		22.4%	77.6%	21.3%	78.7%	33.3%	66.7%
Does the inmate use/abuse drugs?		85.1%	14.9	85.2%	14.8%	83.3%	16.7%
Has inmate been diagnosed with a mental health condition? (51 reported)		15.7%	84.3%	11.5%	67.2%	16.7%	33.3%

Caution is important in interpreting data for women as group is small. Inmates did not always complete all demographic items. All reported above, except last row, had 60 or greater responses total.
s.d. = standard deviation
DNR = did not respond

fluence occupational behavior, and therefore, can prove to also be factors in dysfunctional occupational patterns of behavior.

Clients are provided with a list of statements about occupational functioning, and assess their level of ability when participating in the occupation and their value for that occupation. The OSA assessment uses a two-part self-rating scale. The first section involves a series of statements that review their perceptions of their occupational functioning providing categories for each area as a 'strength,' 'adequate functioning,' or 'weakness.' In the second section, the importance of each of these areas of functioning is also rated. The second section utilizes a similar format but asks the person to rate their environments. Last, the person then prioritizes his or her needs to develop goals and intervention strategies. The last section will not be reported here.

The OSA was built on the results of previous studies of the *Self Assessment of Occupational Functioning* (SAOF) and international studies that sought to reduce culture bias in the instrument (Baron et al., 1999; Henry, 1999). Kielhofner and Forsyth (2001) used Rasch analysis to analyze data from over three hundred physically, psychiatrically or non-disabled adults and reported preliminary validity and reliability of the OSA assessment. Inter-rater reliability for the OSA is not applicable since this is a self-administered assessment. Test-retest reliability has not been reported in published settings though the authors of the OSA suggest that the tool can be appropriate for detecting change in clients (Baron et al., 1999). The latest version of the OSA (Baron, Kielhofner, Iyenger, Goldhammer, & Wolenski, 2002) includes all the same items from the version used in this study. The primary difference is that the response categories in the more recent version have been slightly reworded and expanded from three categories to four to enhance the sensitivity of the instrument. In 2000, when this collaborative study began, the newer version was not available.

Procedures

All OSA evaluations were administered by an occupational therapist (Practice-Scholar) during the intake phase of the project. Demographic information was gathered from the inmate as well as jail records. The standardized protocol for this self-report assessment was used and all were individually administered in the jail in quiet area, typically in the projects classroom area.

RESULTS

The results from the *Occupational Self Assessment* (OSA) are presented in Tables 2 and 3. Each table contains both the self-assessment of occupational functioning with the reported importance. Table 2 reports the findings from total group data analysis (n = 67).

Tables 3 and 4 report the OSA information according to gender. From the beginning of this project, leading staff in the jail reported that woman are not incarcerated as quickly as men for crimes as few judges wish to send women to jail especially since this means separation from their children. As a consequence, women who were incarcerated in jail were reported by staff to have much greater criminal histories than men. Likewise, in occupational therapy, we would conjecture different roles and function between men and women so reporting this additional table seemed appropriate. For example, Jose-Kampfner (2004) reported that up to 80% of incarcerated women are mothers and the role of mothering for these women is clearly influenced by the occupational deprivation inherent in the correctional context. However, caution in using the data in Table 4 is appropriate due to the small *n*.

Difference scores were calculated to determine the disparity between reported occupational competence and the relative importance of the specific occupation to the individual. Those with the highest positive scores are the areas where the competence in performing a given occupation is low compared to the reported importance of this item to the individual. From an intervention perspective, this information is important to consider when prioritizing plans as a change in these may have a major change in overall occupational abilities.

The difference scores across the 3 tables with the highest positive discrepancies are summarized in Table 5 from highest to lowest among the top 8 identified. A notable trend in the data is that four of the items in the table represent environmental components (place to live and take care of myself, basic things I need to live and take care of myself, things I need to be productive, place where I can be productive) and that only one item (managing my finances) focused on a particular performance skill to develop. From an intervention perspective, this information is important to consider when prioritizing plans as a change in these may have a major change in overall occupational abilities. In fact, the practice scholars quickly recognized that while the initial funding they received for the program placed more emphasis on skill building within the county jail context, the real need was for continuous case management and follow-up in the community to support functional patterns of

TABLE 2. OSA Scores – TOTAL GROUP (n = 67)

Assessment Items	STATS	COMPETENCE	IMPORTANCE	DIFFERENCE
1. Concentrating on my tasks	mean	2.21	2.32	0.11
	s.d.	.645	.531	
2. Physically doing what I need to do	mean	2.27	2.33	0.06
	s.d.	.566	.616	
3. Taking care of the place I live	mean	2.60	2.71	0.11
	s.d.	.632	.458	
4. Taking care of myself	mean	2.52	2.83	0.31
	s.d.	.682	.380	
5. Taking care of others for whom I am responsible	mean	2.30	2.56	0.26
	s.d.	.613	.592	
6. Getting where I need to go	mean	2.03	2.34	0.31
	s.d.	.764	.597	
7. Managing my finances	mean	1.69	2.49	0.80
	s.d.	.701	.504	
8. Managing my basic needs	mean	2.20	2.58	0.38
	s.d.	.661	.529	
9. Expressing myself to others	mean	2.06	1.98	0.08
	s.d.	.756	.712	
10. Getting along with others	mean	2.35	2.08	0.27
	s.d.	.568	.640	
11. Identifying and solving problems	mean	2.03	2.37	0.34
	s.d.	.696	.575	
12. Relaxing and enjoying myself	mean	2.28	2.24	0.04
	s.d.	.692	.634	
13. Getting done what I need to do	mean	2.01	2.50	0.49
	s.d.	.707	.562	
14. Having a satisfying routine	mean	1.88	2.08	0.20
	s.d.	.713	.630	
15. Handling my responsibilities	mean	1.82	2.70	0.88
	s.d.	.716	.463	
16. Being involved as a student, worker, volunteer, and/or family member	mean	2.05	2.48	0.43
	s.d.	.672	.589	
17. Doing activities I like	mean	2.35	2.13	0.22
	s.d.	.648	.553	
18. Working towards my goals	mean	1.78	2.62	0.84
	s.d.	.714	.576	
19. Making decisions based on what I think is important	mean	2.06	2.40	0.34
	s.d.	.736	.553	
20. Accomplishing what I set out to do	mean	1.93	2.52	0.59
	s.d.	.724	.561	
21. Effectively using my abilities	mean	2.10	2.47	0.37
	s.d.	.677	.561	
22. Place to live and take care of myself	mean	2.02	2.84	0.82
	s.d.	.875	.366	
23. Place where I can be productive	mean	1.97	2.55	0.58
	s.d.	.684	.532	
24. Basic things I need to live and take care of myself	mean	2.03	2.75	0.72
	s.d.	.728	.436	
25. Things I need to be productive	mean	1.92	2.55	0.63
	s.d.	.664	.502	
26. People who encourage and support me	mean	2.33	2.34	0.01
	s.d.	.730	.676	
27. People who do things with me	mean	2.11	2.07	0.04
	s.d.	.693	.716	
28. Opportunities to do things I value and like	mean	2.11	2.29	0.18
	s.d.	.611	.584	
29. Places where I can enjoy myself	mean	2.14	2.15	0.01
	s.d.	.609	.654	

TABLE 3. OSA Scores – MEN ONLY (n = 61)

OSA–Occupational Self-Assessment–	Statistics	COMPETENCE	IMPORTANCE	DIFFERENCE
1. Concentrating on my tasks	mean s.d.	2.22 .666	2.30 .530	0.08
2. Physically doing what I need to do	mean s.d.	2.26 .575	2.30 .619	0.04
3. Taking care of the place I live	mean s.d.	2.56 .650	2.70 .462	0.14
4. Taking care of myself	mean s.d.	2.49 .698	2.81 .393	0.32
5. Taking care of others for whom I am responsible	mean s.d.	2.25 .606	2.55 .601	0.30
6. Getting where I need to go	mean s.d.	1.97 .758	2.31 .595	0.34
7. Managing my finances	mean s.d.	1.66 .728	2.51 .504	0.85
8. Managing my basic needs	mean s.d.	2.17 .668	2.56 .534	0.39
9. Expressing myself to others	mean s.d.	2.03 .774	1.97 .736	0.06
10. Getting along with others	mean s.d.	2.33 .572	2.07 .660	0.26
11. Identifying and solving problems	mean s.d.	2.02 .695	2.33 .572	0.31
12. Relaxing and enjoying myself	mean s.d.	2.26 .681	2.25 .654	0.01
13. Getting done what I need to do	mean s.d.	1.98 .719	2.47 .566	0.49
14. Having a satisfying routine	mean s.d.	1.87 .724	2.05 .639	0.18
15. Handling my responsibilities	mean s.d.	1.79 .733	2.67 .475	0.88
16. Being involved as a student, worker, volunteer, and/or family member	mean s.d.	2.00 .670	2.44 .595	0.44
17. Doing activities I like	mean s.d.	2.32 .655	2.21 .569	0.11
18. Working towards my goals	mean s.d.	1.70 .691	2.58 .591	0.88
19. Making decisions based on what I think is important	mean s.d.	2.00 .730	2.36 .550	0.36
20. Accomplishing what I set out to do	mean s.d.	1.87 .718	2.48 .567	0.61
21. Effectively using my abilities	mean s.d.	2.03 .657	2.45 .565	0.42
22. Place to live and take care of myself	mean s.d.	1.97 .870	2.83 .381	0.86
23. Place where I can be productive	mean s.d.	1.93 .666	2.50 .538	0.57
24. Basic things I need to live and take care of myself	mean s.d.	2.00 .719	2.74 .442	0.74
25. Things I need to be productive	mean s.d.	1.90 .630	2.50 .505	0.60
26. People who encourage and support me	mean s.d.	2.32 .725	2.29 .680	0.03
27. People who do things with me	mean s.d.	2.09 .683	2.02 .720	0.07
28. Opportunities to do things I value and like	mean s.d.	2.08 .619	2.27 .556	0.19
29. Places where I can enjoy myself	mean s.d.	2.10 .607	2.11 .658	0.01

TABLE 4. OSA Scores – WOMEN ONLY (n = 6)

OSA - Occupational Self-Assessment -	Statistics	COMPETENCE	IMPORTANCE	DIFFERENCE
1. Concentrating on my tasks	mean s.d.	2.17 .408	2.50 .548	0.33
2. Physically doing what I need to do	mean s.d.	2.33 .516	2.67 .516	0.34
3. Taking care of the place I live	mean s.d.	3.00 0.00	2.80 .447	− 0.20
4. Taking care of myself	mean s.d.	2.83 .408	3.00 .000	0.17
5. Taking care of others for whom I am responsible	mean s.d.	2.83 .408	2.60 .548	0.23
6. Getting where I need to go	mean s.d.	2.67 .516	2.80 .447	0.13
7. Managing my finances	mean s.d.	2.00 .000	2.33 .516	0.33
8. Managing my basic needs	mean s.d.	2.50 .548	2.80 .447	0.30
9. Expressing myself to others	mean s.d.	2.33 .516	2.17 .408	− 0.16
10. Getting along with others	mean s.d.	2.50 .548	2.17 .408	− 0.33
11. Identifying and solving problems	mean s.d.	2.17 .753	2.80 .447	0.63
12. Relaxing and enjoying myself	mean s.d.	2.50 .837	2.17 .408	−0.33
13. Getting done what I need to do	mean s.d.	2.33 .516	2.83 .408	0.50
14. Having a satisfying routine	mean s.d.	2.00 .632	2.33 .516	0.33
15. Handling my responsibilities	mean s.d.	2.17 .408	3.00 0.00	0.83
16. Being involved as a student, worker, volunteer, and/or family member	mean s.d.	2.50 .548	2.83 .408	0.33
17. Doing activities I like	mean s.d.	2.67 .516	2.17 .408	−0.50
18. Working towards my goals	mean s.d.	2.50 .548	3.00 .000	0.50
19. Making decisions based on what I think is important	mean s.d.	2.67 .516	2.83 .408	0.16
20. Accomplishing what I set out to do	mean s.d	2.50 .548	2.83 .408	0.33
21. Effectively using my abilities	mean s.d.	2.83 .408	2.67 .516	0.16
22. Place to live and take care of myself	mean s.d.	2.50 .837	3.00 0.00	0.50
23. Place where I can be productive	mean s.d.	2.33 .816	3.00 0.00	0.67
24. Basic things I need to live and take care of myself	mean s.d.	2.33 .816	2.83 .408	0.50
25. Things I need to be productive	mean s.d.	2.17 .983	3.00 0.00	0.83
26. People who encourage and support me	mean s.d.	2.50 .837	2.83 .408	0.33
27. People who do things with me	mean s.d.	2.33 .816	2.50 .548	0.17
28. Opportunities to do things I value and like	mean s.d.	2.33 .516	2.50 .837	0.17
29. Places where I can enjoy myself	mean s.d.	2.50 .548	2.50 .548	0

occupation. Subsequent funding requests emphasized the process of community reintegration with a heavy emphasis on developing the environmental supports necessary to maintain community living. Due to the small number, a "*" is used to indicate ones for women that are similar with men.

The other two categories that showed the greatest divergence for women were: 'identifying and solving problems' and 'getting done what I need to do.' One can see that time management, productive goal setting, contexts to support occupations and managing finances are critical occupational issues.

DISCUSSION

This case study has served two purposes: (1) to overview the value of an academic-practice partnership that is demonstrating the potential to engage in the successful scholarship of practice to provide evidence to support the role of occupational therapy in jails; and (2) using systematic approaches to evaluation to embed research into daily practice activities that accumulated over time can provide guidance in program planning as well as document information useful to support OT practice in a given area.

As more systematic data is collected on this population using this OSA, additional questions will be explored. For instance, do inmates who were rated as successful in our program differ in initial OSA scores than those who were not? Does occupational disruption and needs change based on the number of re-incarcerations? What types of environmental interventions or supports are most effective in reducing recidivism? How do differences in demographic variables relate to

TABLE 5. Rank Order of Highest Competence-Value Difference Scores

	Total	Men	Women
	(n = 67)	(n = 61)	(n = 6)
Handling my responsibilities	.88	.88	*
Working towards my goals	.84	.88	*
Place to live and take care of myself	.82	.86	*
Managing my finances	.80	.85	
Basic things I need to live and take care of myself	.72	.74	*
Things I need to be productive	.62	.60	*
Accomplishing what I set out to do	.59	.61	
Place where I can be productive	.58	.57	*

differences in occupational adaptation? And of course, the most critical one that requires re-test data–does the community integration program described here positively influence or change occupational competence and/or result in sustained community re-integration?

The role and function of occupational therapy in the jail is an incredible opportunity. The populations are increasing exponentially and recidivism is the major issue, as seen in this case study. With the goal of release in less than two years, the need to learn healthier occupational patterns and habits is essential to lower recidivism, increase, occupational productivity and quality of life among released inmates, and ultimately protect the public by lowering crime. Certainly, occupational therapy enhanced through academic-practice partnerships can provide extraordinary activities that promote the profession through the scholarship of practice and demonstrate a valuable, productive engagement between faculty and practitioners.

REFERENCES

Baron, K. (1991). *The Self Assessment of Occupational Functioning: An efficacy study.* Unpublished master's thesis, University of Illinois at Chicago.

Baron, K. B. & Curtin, C. (1990). *A manual for use with the Self Assessment of Occupational Functioning.* Department of Occupational Therapy, University of Illinois at Chicago.

Baron, K., Kielhofner, G., Goldhammer, V., & Wolenski, J. (1999). *The Occupational Self Assessment (OSA) (Version 1.0).* Chicago: Model of Human Occupation Clearinghouse, Department of Occupational Therapy, College of Applied Health Sciences, University of Illinois at Chicago.

Baron, K., Kielhofner, G., Iyenger, A., Goldhammer, V., & Wolenski, J. (2002). *The Occupational Self Assessment (OSA) (Version 2.0).* Chicago: Model of Human Occupation Clearinghouse, Department of Occupational Therapy, College of Applied Health Sciences, University of Illinois at Chicago.

Benson, B. L. (1998). *To serve and protect: Privatization and community in criminal justice.* New York: New York University Press.

Cara, E. & MacRae, A. (2005). *Psychosocial Occupational Therapy: A Clinical Practice (2 ed.).* Albany, NY: Delmar Publishers.

Department of Justice, Bureau of Statistics, *"Prison and Jail Inmates at Midyear 2002"* (April 6, 2003). Retrieved January 27, 2004 from *http://www.ojp.usdojgov/bjs/abstract/pjim02.htm*

Dressler, J. & Snively, F. (1998). Occupational therapy in the criminal justice system. In E. Cara & A. McRae (Eds.) *Psychosocial occupational therapy: A clinical practice* (pp. 527-552). Albany: Delmar Publishers.

Eggers, M., Muñoz, J. P., Sciulli, J., & Crist, P. A. (Submitted for review) The Community Reintegration Project: Occupational Therapy at Work in a County Jail. *Occupational Therapy in Health Care.*

Eggers, M., Scuilli, J., Gauguzis, K., & Muñoz, J. P. (2003, June). Enrichment through occupation: The Allegheny County Jail Project. *AOTA Mental Health Special Interest Quarterly, 26* (2), 1-4.

Greenfeld, L. (1985). Examining Recidivism. Bureau of Justice Statistics Special Report. Washington, D.C.: U.S. Department of Justice, Bureau of Justice Statistics.

Henry, A. D., Baron, K. B., Mouradian, L., & Curtin, C. (1999). Reliability and validity of the self-assessment of occupational functioning. *American Journal of Occupational Therapy, 53* (5), 482-488.

Jones, E. J. & McColl, M. A. (1991). Development and evaluation of an interaction life skills group of offenders. *The Occupational Therapy Journal of Research*, 11, 80-92.

Jose-Kampfner, C. (2004). Mothering from prison: It can be done! In S. A. Esdaile & J. A. Olson (eds.), *Mothering occupations: Challenge, agency and participation* (pp. 259-281. Philadelphia: F. A. Davis.

Keilhofner, G. (2002). *Model of human occupation: Theory and application*, 3rd ed. Baltimore: Lippincott, Williams, & Wilkins.

Kielhofner, G. & Forsyth, K. (2001). Measurement properties of a client self-report for treatment planning and documenting therapy outcomes. *Scandinavian Journal of Occupational Therapy 8* (3), 131-139.

Lederer, J., Kielhofner, G., & Watts, J. (1985). Values, personal causation and skills of delinquents and nondelinquents. *Occupational Theory in Mental Health*, 5 (2), 59-77.

Needles, K. (1996). Go directly to jail and do not collect? A long-term study of recidivism, employment, and earnings among prison releases. *Journal of Crime and Delinquency*, 33 (4), 471-496.

Petersilia, J. (2000). When prisoners return to the community: Political, economic, and social consequences. Sentencing and Corrections: Issues for the 21st Century. Washington, DC: U.S. Department of Justice, Office of Justice Programs, November 2000. Retrieved from *www.ncjrs.org/pdffiles1/nij/184253.pdf* on December 16, 2004.

Scaffa, M. (2001). *Occupational therapy in community-based practice settings*. Philadelphia: F. A. Davis.

Wilcock, A. (1998). *An occupational perspective of health*. Thorofare, NJ: Slack.

Achieving Evidence-Based Practice:
A Process of Continuing Education
Through Practitioner-Academic Partnership

Kirsty Forsyth, PhD, OTR
Jane Melton, MSc, DipCOT
Lynn Summerfield Mann, MSc, DipCOT

Kirsty Forsyth is Director, UK Centre for Outcomes Research and Education (UKCORE), London South Bank University, London; and Senior Lecturer at the Queen Margaret University College, Edinburgh. Jane Melton is Consultant Occupational Therapist, Gloucestershire Partnership NHS Trust, Cheltenham, England. Lynn Summerfield Mann is Principle Lecturer, Occupational Therapy Post Graduate Programme and Co-Director, UK Centre for Outcomes Research and Education (UKCORE), London South Bank University, London.

The authors would like to acknowledge the following stakeholders involved in this UKCORE/GPT partnership: Julia Bowden, John Cooper, Victoria Derrick, Melanie Harrison, Mac McHardy, Andrea Moffatt, Katie Medhurst, Ruth Roberts, Jayne Robinson, Micheline Robson Ward, Karen Rogers, Laura Wain, are all occupational therapists who have had a role in pioneering this educational development.

Tricia Larrett and Jill Lucas are occupational therapy leaders within the GPT who have contributed expert knowledge to support and resource this development.

[Haworth co-indexing entry note]: "Achieving Evidence-Based Practice: A Process of Continuing Education Through Practitioner-Academic Partnership." Forsyth, Kirsty, Jane Melton, and Lynn Summerfield Mann. Co-published simultaneously in *Occupational Therapy in Health Care* (The Haworth Press, Inc.) Vol. 19, No. 1/2, 2005, pp. 211-227; and: *The Scholarship of Practice: Academic-Practice Collaborations for Promoting Occupational Therapy* (ed: Patricia Crist, and Gary Kielhofner) The Haworth Press, Inc., 2005, pp. 211-227. Single or multiple copies of this article are available for a fee from The Haworth Document Delivery Service [1-800-HAWORTH, 9:00 a.m.-5:00 p.m. (EST). E-mail address: docdelivery@haworthpress.com].

Available online at http://www.haworthpress.com/web/OTHC
doi:10.1300/J003v19n01_15

SUMMARY. Occupational therapy is required to deliver and generate evidence-based practice. As currently articulated, evidence-based practice requires particular skills and takes time and is rarely realized. This paper illustrates a collaborative approach to building an evidence based training program within a practice context. The aim of the training program was to enable therapists in a large mental health setting to engage in evidence-based practice. Specifically, the partnership between the United Kingdom Centre for Outcomes Research and Education (UK CORE) and Gloucestershire Partnership NHS Trust (GPT) will be described. This article describes the GPT/UKCORE partnership, the process of building an evidence-based practice training program, the final structure of the evidence-based practice training program, and the evaluation of the evidence-based practice training program. *[Article copies available for a fee from The Haworth Document Delivery Service: 1-800-HAWORTH. E-mail address: <docdelivery@haworthpress.com> Website: <http://www.HaworthPress.com> © 2005 by The Haworth Press, Inc. All rights reserved.]*

KEYWORDS. Continuing education, theory use, evidence-based practice

BACKGROUND AND RATIONALE

Evidence-based practice has been defined as the judicious use of the best available evidence to guide decision making in health care (Sackett et al., 1996). The Health Industry is increasingly demanding that occupational therapists deliver evidence-based practice (Lloyd et al., 2004). Consequently, for occupational therapy to remain valued, it is essential for the profession to adopt an evidence-based approach to practice delivery (McCluskey & Cusick, 2002). Delivering and generating evidence-based practice, however, poses significant challenges in practical settings (SEHD, 2002).

Practicing therapists appear to agree with the necessity of evidence-based practice, since they consistently report a belief that research and theory is important to guide practice (Metcalfe et al., 2001; Humphries et al., 2000; Bennett et al., 2003). Despite therapists' willingness, it appears that they often lack the skill and knowledge to change practice based on evidence (NHS Centre for Reviews and Dissemination, 1999). Evidence-based practice requires knowledge about research and how to critique as well as the wherewithal to subsequently know how to synthesize evidence into one's daily work routine (MacEwan, Dysart, &

Tomlin 2002; Bennett et al., 2003; Humphries et al., 2000). Post qualification training has been identified as a potential mechanism for gaining these skills, moreover in the UK and elsewhere post qualification education is expected or mandated for practitioners (COT, 2004) and is necessary to ensure ongoing registration/licensure. However, there is evidence that therapists do not have the skills and habits to implement evidence-based practice despite post qualification education requirements and opportunities (NHS Centre for Reviews and Dissemination, 1999; Roberts, 2002). It appears, then, that traditional post qualification education has not effectively addressed the barriers to evidence-based practice that therapists encounter in their daily practice.

Traditional evidence-based training programs (EBPP) have been developed by academics. An alternative collaborative approach between academia and practice will be presented. This article will describe the GPT/UKCORE partnership, process of building an evidence-based practice training program, the final structure of the evidence-based practice training program, and the evaluation of the evidence-based practice training program. These are discussed below.

GLOUCESTERSHIRE PARTNERSHIP NHS TRUST (GPT)/UKCORE PARTNERSHIP

In April 2002, the Gloucestershire Partnership NHS Trust (GPT) was formed following significant organizational change in health and social care services in England, UK. GPT is a specialist National Health Service (NHS) organization that delivers services for people with Mental Illness and those with Learning Disabilities. GPT is committed to transforming health and social care provision for its service users and considers it vital to develop and maintain the highest clinical standards (Gloucestershire Health Authority 2001). The second author approached UKCORE to work in partnership with the occupational therapy service in order to develop and enhance the routine use of evidence-based practice.

The UKCORE was originally built on the principles from scholarship of practice (Kielhofner, in press). UKCORE set out 3 years ago to integrate scholarship (i.e., research and theory development), education, and practice. The UKCORE now involves ongoing relationships with five groups of therapists located in different health organizations throughout England and Scotland, one of which is GPT.

GPT and UKCORE have been working in partnership together for two years and have been delivering and generating evidence-based practice. One aspect of this partnership has been the development of an evidence-based practice (EBP) educational programme for qualified therapists. The following section discusses how the EBP programme was developed.

Process of Building Evidence-Based Practice Training Programme

As previously discussed, practitioners tend not to have access to strategically planned and systematically provided post qualification education that addressed the real challenges of integrating evidence into practice (NHS Centre for Reviews and Dissemination, 1999). The partnership wanted to develop an EBP training program within the organization that responded to how therapists perceived their needs. This meant that a great deal of attention had to been paid to understanding the situation and in order to create graded, specific educational experiences that reflected local needs.

The approach to rethinking how to tackle the EBP training program was action research (AR) (Taylor, Braveman, & Hammel, in press; Kielhofner, Hammel, Helfrich, Finlayson, & Taylor, in press; Tewey, 1997; Jason et al., 2003). This approach allows those who ultimately use the training to be involved in helping to generate and refine it, the development of the post registration education needs to be grounded in the context in which it is designed, and it should emerge from cooperation and teamwork between those whose traditional role it is to complete training and those whose roles involve applying this knowledge in practice. Consequently, AR calls for a dynamic collaboration between researchers and all the key stakeholders in the setting where the continuing education takes place. The action research strategy was a phased approach involving problem identification, building an implementation plan, and evaluation. This approach allowed for the identification of why previous educational opportunities had not supported evidence-based changes in practice. Moreover, it was responsive to how therapists perceived their needs, challenges and barriers. This ensured practice stakeholders were part of the process of finding an appropriate content and format for the training.

Problem Identification

Problem identification focused on bringing all the stakeholders together to collect and analyse data on the previous methods of training. In order to obtain the perspective of qualified colleagues around their

EBP training needs and what form this training should take, academics and practitioners engaged in a joint process of participatory visioning.

A group reflective approach was taken to identify the challenges of previous methods of training. This information, once analysed, could support the building of a new training solution. Therefore, representatives of the GPT therapists engaged in dialogue with academics from the UKCORE. This involved academics using open ended questions to facilitate therapists to process their previous educational experiences and support them to formulate for themselves, their vision of their needs and how they wanted them addressed. The initial group consensus identified many problems with the traditional approaches to post qualification education (see Table 1). These were clustered into issues of (i) Content of educational programme, (ii) Structure of Educational Programme.

(i) Content of Educational Programme

Use of New Knowledge in Practice. It was identified that previous education lacked information on how to use new knowledge in practice. The traditional approach could have involved GPT in negotiating for

TABLE 1. Problem Identification

Problem Identified	Specific Issue
Content of Educational Programme	
Difficulty *using* new knowledge in practice	Didactic sessions provided to increase knowledge, but no specific support from "experts" to use knowledge in practice
Content of EBP training	Colleagues overwhelmed by the topic and wanted it broken down into smaller "subtopics"
Educational Style	Didactic teaching was not always appropriate and more effective ways of engaging colleagues in an educational process was required.
Structure of Educational Programme	
Lack of access of some colleagues to educational sessions	UKCORE "experts" attended a limited number of sessions Part time colleagues, illness or maternity leave were all identified as reasons for not being able to attend Lack of finance for more UKCORE sessions
Colleague attrition	Colleagues join and leave a service over time OT is not an evidence-based profession and therefore new colleagues joining won't have EBP skills Need for ongoing EBP educational opportunities
Role definition	Practitioners holding trainer roles would provide more opportunities for colleagues to access an ongoing programme Trainer roles would be new to practitioners and support would be needed

UKCORE colleagues to deliver didactic training sessions. These sessions would have focused on building knowledge about EBP and would not have discussed how to use this knowledge when therapists went back to their workplaces. This is reflective of traditional training whereby visiting "educators" provide information on a specific topic, then they leave, with the therapists being left to apply the new knowledge on their own. This can lead to high levels of frustration within the service because colleagues were exposed to new ideas on how to develop their practice but find it very challenging to deliver this new knowledge in their work places.

Topics Within EBP Training. Colleagues also reported they were feeling overwhelmed by the evidence-based agenda. The topic is broad and therapist requested it be phased in order to build knowledge incrementally. It was felt that it would be appropriate to follow the OT process and start the education with evidence-based assessment. It was also acknowledged that one evidence-based assessment would not be appropriate for all practice areas and a range of evidence-based assessment training would be required (see Table 2).

Educational Style. Information from previous training opportunities had identified the importance of the experiences within the training. The

TABLE 2. Content and Format of Sessions

Session 1	
Content	**Format**

Learn new EBP knowledge
  National/local context for EBP
  Knowing how to choose between EB
  assessments
  Becoming familiar with administration and scoring
  of EB assessment
	Lecture
	Interactive discussion
	Small group work
	Viewing of video cases
	Problem solving
	Role play
	Case studies

How to implement new knowledge in workplace
  Thinking through practical implications of service changes
  How to socially negotiate with multidisciplinary team
  EB changes that affect them
  Review of work routines and how time is spent
  How to reconstruct routine to support EB changes
  Consider support mechanisms
  Goal setting	

3 months between session 1 & 2	
Session 2	
Content	**Format**

Experiences of using EBP knowledge in practice
  Sharing of experiences
  Problem solving around challenges experienced
  Review of goals set in session 1
  Set new goals
	Peer case studies
	Interactive discussion
	Problem solving

training sessions needed to be engaging and enjoyable. Participants needed to feel involved and active in the session and particularly found benefit from a range of educational methods, e.g., including basic information on the EBP topic, case studies to illustrate the EBP topic from a peer within the clinical organisation, and role playing to practice EBP skills.

(ii) Structure of Educational Programme

Access to Training. There were concerns raised around how to improve training opportunities for therapists who were not able to attend the UKCORE led sessions. Part of the colleagues group reported they felt disadvantaged by not being able to access the training sessions and a desire was expressed that all colleagues needed equal access to post qualification training. Having a larger number of UKCORE lead sessions would accommodate all colleagues, however, this would require more finances. Having external educators routinely visit to complete education would be expensive. Therapists, therefore, identified that they needed regular session lead by GPT colleagues. This would keep costs down and provide a routine mechanism to deliver the training. (NHS Centre for Reviews and Dissemination, 1999; FoNS, 2001).

Colleague Attrition. Colleagues feedback also identified that there was an issue with natural attrition of colleagues. Colleagues joined and left the services for a range of reasons and therefore there was a natural turnover of colleagues within the services. Concerns were identified that the profession in general was not yet evidence-based and therefore new colleagues joining the organization would not necessarily be bringing this knowledge and skills with them. They would therefore need support to gain EBP knowledge and skills. This reinforced the conclusion that there was a need for ongoing training over time.

Role Definition. The traditional approach involved GPT negotiating for UKCORE colleagues to deliver didactic training sessions. This is reflective of traditional training whereby visiting "educators" provide information on a specific topic. The consensus of the group lead to the acknowledgment that any new educational structure needed to change traditional roles. Rather, than the academics holding the "educational" role and practitioners holding the "student" role, a new system of relationships was envisioned with people taking newly defined roles and activities. Specifically, this means that practitioners take on the trainer role with support from the academic "experts." This would allow a practice-based training programme to be developed that would meet the needs of the service and be financially viable. The trainer role would be a new responsibility for most of the practitioners and, therefore, peer feedback and support was seen as essential.

The development of the implementation plan needed to therefore address both issues of content and structure of the educational program. The advantage of this dual approach would allow the delivery of practice based educational session within a broader educational structure. It was hoped by addressing the above concerns the educational programme would both increase therapists' knowledge and skills in areas of identified need, and embed this knowledge and skill into the routines of everyday clinical life. This dual strategy allows the building of therapist's capacity to be able to deliver evidence-based practice more consistently within the clinical setting.

Implementation Plan

Practical issues of developing a program in terms of content and structure needed to be addressed during the planning process. These are discussed below.

(i) Content of Educational Programme

Use of New Knowledge in Practice. In order to respond to the therapists' difficulty of not "knowing" how to put the new knowledge into practice, supportive strategies were identified. Creating educational content that included not only learning new EBP knowledge, but also how to plan the implementation of this knowledge in practice was completed. This included how to negotiate with multi disciplinary teams to integrate an evidence-based change in practice which may affect team members, how to review work routines to accommodate new evidence-based procedures, how to obtain support through supervision and from peers, etc.

Topics Within EBP Training. In order to ensure the topic of evidence-based practice was approached in a graded way, it was decided to follow the OT process. The initial focus, therefore, was on evidence-based assessment. The content of these sessions were identified as the identification of the most appropriate EB assessment, learning how to administer it in a reliable and valid manner, completing rater reliability testing, how to formulate cases from the assessment findings, etc.

In order to further facilitate a graded approach, a series of two sessions were chosen. The first session would focus on introductory information. Learning outcomes for the first session were focused to facilitate an understanding of the national and local context for evidence-based practice, develop knowledge and skills around the topic of the session, and formulate personal goals and action plan for re-entering the workplace. A very clear message of the session was identified as all OTs were expected to deliver evidence-based services and it is each OTs responsibility to ensure they have the right kinds of supports to be able to achieve this overall goal.

The second session was timed to be three months later to allow time for the participants to use the information from the first session in their clinical setting and attempt to reach their stated goals. The content of the second session was focused on sharing of experiences, problem solving around challenges that arose in practice, review of goals and identify if goals were not achieved and if not, why not. Issues would be identified prior to the session so that there could be preparation around specific concerns.

Educational Style. The initial problem identification highlighted that colleagues appreciated a range of educational methods and didn't find a didactic approach alone sufficient for understanding the information being shared. The sessions were, therefore, focused on providing various educational experiences and support (Gerrish & Clayton, 2004; Humphries et al., 2000). These include lecture format, interactive discussion forums, small group work, viewing of videos, sharing of clinical experiences, doing evidence-based practice, reporting out of assessments, proactive problem solving around fears and anxieties, role playing situations that required social negotiation to allow for EBP, and identification of implications for management support. These techniques were all supportive of the expectation that participants would return to practice and apply their learning. This would form a major part of the learning process. Participants were held to account for this in their follow-up training session and via ongoing clinical supervision.

(ii) Structure of Educational Programme

Access to Training. The decision to support practitioners to become trainers increased the number of colleagues within the organization who had specialist evidence-based practice skill. The partners felt it would be important to have practitioners representing all service areas in the trust involved in training roles. These areas included adult mental health, older people's mental health, child and family services, and services for people with learning disabilities. This would ensure that all practice areas had specified trainers and would ensure each practice area had access to a trainer. Timings and frequency of session were considered carefully to ensure there was coverage across the colleagues group to allow for equal access of all members of colleagues to the training.

Consideration was also given to how to recruit colleagues' members to the educational sessions. It was felt that a large number of OTs would want to take up this new educational opportunity and a transparent process of access was needed. Moreover, the trainers expressed an interest in supporting the therapists to be prepared for the sessions. Prerequisites for the sessions were, therefore, identified. For example, the course participants needed to be: qualified members of colleagues, have evidence-based skill building identified in their individual development plans, have already attended general EBP induction, have completed some background reading on the topic, and be able to commit to the series of sessions. This allowed the appropriate group of therapists to be identified through a transparent process. There was a process of identifying and recruiting colleagues to the sessions. Parameters around the number of participants and the frequency of sessions were identified and this allowed an estimate of the time it would take to educate the entire service. These structures were perceived by the practice educators to put boundaries around the initiative and therefore made the implementation more manageable.

Colleagues' Attrition. The educational programme was constructed to have both regular induction sessions and ongoing EBP assessment training sessions. This was specifically to ensure all colleagues would receive EBP education as they joined the service. The induction session was focused on the evidence based expectations of the service and an orientation to the specific requirement of them as a therapist within the service. Every new member of colleagues needs to attend an induction session within 4 weeks of arriving. The regularity of the evidence-based assessment training allowed for new members of colleagues to receive this training early in their new position.

Role Definition

Identifying and supporting trainers would be the most important aspect of the program. The role of a trainer was outlined and specific benefits of being a trainer were identified as including improved knowledge of evidence-based practice principles and assessments, improved skill to identify appropriate EB assessments for different practice areas, and developed ability to critique EB assessments. This provided an increased overall understanding of evidence-based practice *choices* and how these choices can be made systematically. Moreover, leadership skills were developed within these roles. The trainers would be expected to have more advanced knowledge than other therapists and be able to guide and support other therapists to make their own appropriate evidence-based decisions.

Identifying Trainers

It is worthy to note that this style of disseminating best, evidence-based practice has no shortage of occupational therapist recruits to the trainer role. The enthusiasm of the trainers towards this initiative is contagious and has led to a successful programme of practice development being founded. The trainer specifications allowed potential trainers to match the new knowledge and skills built through their participation in this new role with career objectives. Several therapists saw this as an opportunity to build EB skills to be able to present more clearly within their multi-disciplinary team. The confidence that comes from knowing an EB assessment in detail and presenting case studies routinely in the training session were seen as transferable skills into their own practice when presenting cases to their multidisciplinary team. Other therapists saw this as an opportunity to build EB skills to be able to undertake lecturing at a local OT continuing education programme in addition to being an opportunity to strengthen their EB skill to support student education within the practice context.

Clinicians who had recognized in their personal development plans that they wanted to develop educational skills were contacted. Therapists who had natural leadership qualities were also sought. The individual therapists, who were identified as having well developed evidence based skills were validated by this perception of their ability. This lead them to reflect on their skills and obtain a more accurate sense of their abilities. An example of this is a colleague who would typically not volunteer to present work has become increasingly respected for their contribution to practice teaching. Therapists of various senior grades were asked through clinical supervision to participate. Though sometimes expressing that this was initially daunting, volunteers saw this as an excellent opportunity to develop both their clinical and their leadership skills.

Trainer Meetings to Support Role Development

Having a meeting structure allowed trainers to have access to service leaders, academics and their peer trainers have, over time, developed further confidence and skill in their contribution to this role (see Figure 1). The trainers were excited about this new role, however, did express some anxieties at being seen as evidence-based "experts" within the organisation. There was, therefore, discussion around the specific concerns and potential supports. For instance, the first course participants were selected carefully so that they would be supportive of the trainers' new role, trainers were supported to answer questions in a role playing situation, and support would be provided from UKCORE and OT leaders to develop the educational materials. It was identified that confidence could also be supported by the trainers having access to "EBP experts" from UKCORE. In order to provide "expert" support the trainers were part of a larger group with UKCORE to form the "education team" for the organisation (see Figure 2). Regular meetings of this team were focused around how to bring the individual EB assessment session into a structure that would support the ongoing success of the initiative. This group discussed general implementation issues and produced the organisational action plan.

The partnership wanted to support these trainers as much as possible to deliver education around EB assessments. It was identified in the literature that encouraging clinicians to work in small groups may help to maintain motivation and provide practical support (Conroy, 1997). The trainers were therefore organised into small groups of three leaders according to the specific assessment that they were leading on (see Figure 2). This provided the trainers with peer support around the specific assessment they were leading on. The trainers found it helpful to have support from others who were charged with the same responsibility. Peer feedback and support was seen as essential by individuals to support the education delivery. Having more than one trainer for each assessment

FIGURE 1. Peer Meetings

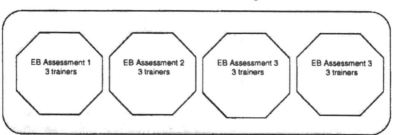

Note: Each evidence-based assessment has 3 trainers. Each group of three trainers meet to discuss the implementation of the EB assessment they are responsible for.

FIGURE 2. All EB Assessment Groups Meet Together with UKCORE

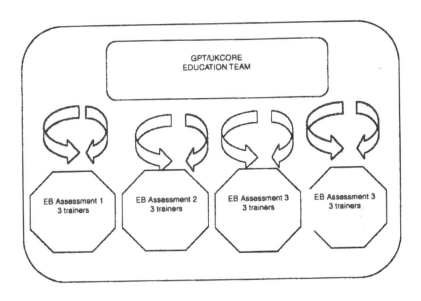

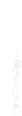

allowed for peer support and also provided a framework to support for illness, maternity leave, and trainers leaving the organisation. This meeting monitored the progress of the initiative. The challenges of delivering the program can be discussed at this meeting and solutions found. Strategic planning around dissemination of the success of the program can also be done through this group. Initially the trainers wanted to develop a strong cohesive support group as the priority and this group would then be used more as a monitoring and evaluation group as the initiative matured.

Time to Deliver Trainer Role

The ongoing dialogue focused around the development of specific supports to tackle the logistics of having a robust EBP training component delivered in an efficient way. Time and competing priorities are often cited as important barriers to the success of initiatives like this (Humphries, 1998). OTs were concerned about how they would be able to meet the responsibilities of this extra trainer role. Therefore, sequestered time for trainers was identified to allow for the development and management of the training programme.

Supporting Accountability as a Trainer

It was also felt that therapists should be held accountable for integration of this knowledge through supervision structures. Accountability in any system is important. It was felt strongly by the trainers that the service needed to embed the new knowledge and skills gained in the sessions. An accountability system was therefore required to ensure that this was taking place. Through partnership discussion it was decided that participants should write departmental and personal goals as part of the educational experience. In addition to this, each participant was expected to attend a follow-up session where these goals would be monitored. Other mechanisms were identified for monitoring, for example, goals would be shared with individuals' clinical supervisors so that supervisors could support the participants' process. Trainers held a hard copy of all goals and goals achieved to allow for overall monitoring to occur.

EVALUATION

All partners wanted to ensure that everyone in the service knew the success of the initiative. There was careful partnership dialogue around how OTs would know if the programme was supportive of developing EBP knowledge/skills and if this translated into the changing of practice to be more evidence based. Several mechanisms were identified as being indicators of success. These are described in Figure 3.

Self-Report Evaluation. Changing practice is a collaborative venture (Humphries, 1998) so consumers of initiatives need to be consulted about their experience and identify what was supportive of their learning and practice changes. Self-report evaluation forms were designed for participants to complete on the day. These can then be analysed to allow feedback to the individual trainers and aggregated as an indicator of the overall success of the initiative.

Trainer Reflections. It was also felt important for individual trainers to be reflective about their skills. Reflection is central to the art of good practice (Roberts, 2002; Schon, 1991). Part of the evaluation was, therefore, based on the principles and values associated with practice reflection. Its purpose is to promote self-knowledge, personal development and confidence. It also ensures that developmental and training needs are identified. There are individual levels of ability to reflect on leadership skills. Reflection structures are provided for those who want more structure around their

FIGURE 3. Evaluation of Education

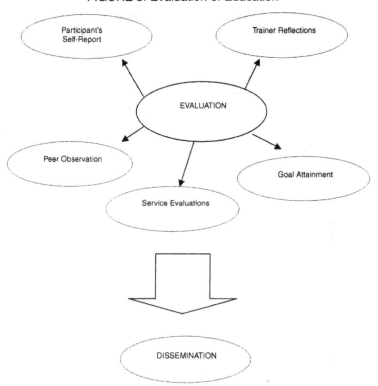

reflections. These reflections can be shared in the educational leaders group or with individual mentors within the organization.

Peer Observation, It was felt that learning from each other via peer observation would also be an important benefit in the project development (Sleep et al., 2002). Peer evaluation forms were developed to allow other leaders to view the session and provide constructive feedback about the performance of the people facilitating the session. The peer evaluation is divided into three parts. First, there is preparation for the observation. This is a brief meeting before the session so that the peer observer can discuss the educational leaders overall objectives and learning outcomes for the session. The observation is recorded in a standard format and feedback is provided after the session. The written feedback can then be used to inform future sessions, in supervision with a mentor, or develop action points to take to the larger education group.

Service Evaluation. Feedback might also be obtained from some of the other evidence-based structures that are already in place. The service already completes a service evaluation of their evidence-based activities. The educational component can be built into this preexisting evaluation procedures. For example, evidence-based meetings throughout the organisation have already been established to support problem solving. These meetings can have an agenda item eliciting comments on the usefulness of the educational component to the organization's activities.

Goal Attainment. Participants will be asked to set departmental and personal goals in the first session and this will be monitored. A statement can therefore be made about the percentage of goals that have been achieved.

Dissemination. Dissemination of success was also considered. The GPT/UKCORE annual report would identify the success in the year including the educational component. This will include a write-up of the range of the evaluations completed. Other communication strategies will be used to promote the educational program and its importance to continued professional development. For example, the clinical educators have developed a sense of new found confidence and courage to plan conference presentations based on their innovative work.

CONCLUSION

This paper describes a collaborative partnership that supported a clinical group to develop an educational strategy to embed evidence-based practice into clinical life. A set of dialogues and negotiations were exchanged to allow for the building of an educational structure to support the initiative. Each partner brought their own views and belief to the negotiations and a shared view was developed. The resulting educational program was embedded within practice and focused on improving knowledge of evidence based practice and how to make evidence-based practice changes within the realities of clinical life.

REFERENCES

Bennett, S., Tooth, L., McKenna, K., Rodger, S., Strong, J., Ziviani, J., Mickan. S., & Gibson, L. (2003). *Australian Journal of Occupational Therapy*, 50, 13-22.

Conroy, M. (1997). "Why are you doing that?" A project to look for evidence of efficacy within occupational therapy. *British Journal of Occupational Therapy*, 60, 487-490.

Fitzgerland, L., Ferlie, E., & Hawkins, C. (2003). Innovations in healthcare: How does credible evidence influence professionals? *Health and Social Care in the Community, 11 (3) 219-228.*

Foundation of Nursing Studies (2001). *Taking Action: Moving towards evidence-based practice*. London: FoNS.

Gerish, K., and Clayton J. (2004). Promoting evidence-based practice: An organisational approach. *Journal of Nursing Management* 12, 114-123.

Gloucestershire Health Authority (2001). "Meeting the Challenge–Proposals for Developing Health Services in Gloucestershire, Consultation Document."

HEFCE (2001). *Promoting research in nursing and the allied health professions*. Report to Task group 3.

Humphries, D. (1998). Managing knowledge into practice. *Manual Therapy* 3 (3) 153-158.

Humphries, D., Littlejohns P., Victor C., O'Halloran P., & Peacock J. (2000). Implementing Evidence-Based Practice: Factors that Influence the Use of Research Evidence by Occupational Therapists. *British Journal of Occupational Therapy*, 63 (11) 516-522.

Kaner, E., Steven, A., Cassidy, P., & Vardy, C. (2005). Implementation of a model for service delivery and organisation in mental healthcare: A qualitative exploration of service provider views, *Health and Social Care in the Community*, 11 (6) 519-527.

Kielhofner, G. (2005) Scholarship and Practice: Bridging the divide. *American Journal of Occupational Therapy*, 59, 231-239.

Kielhofner, G., Hammel, J., Helfrich, C., Finlayson, M., & Taylor, R. (2004). Studying practice and its outcomes: A conceptual approach. *American Journal of Occupational Therapy*, 58, 15-23.

Lloyd, C., Basset, H., & King, R. (2004). Occupational Therapy and evidence-based practice in mental health, *British Journal of Occupational Therapy*, 67 (2) p. 83-88.

Locock, L., Dopson, S., Chamber, D.,& Gabbay, J. (2001) Understanding opinion leaders roles. *Social Science and Medicine* 53, 745-757.

McCluskey, A., & Cusick, A. (2002). Strategies for introducing evidence-based practice and changing clinical behaviour: A managers toolbox, *Australian Occupational Therapy Journal* 49, 63-70.

Metcalf, C., Perry, S., Bannigan, K., Lewin, R. J. P., Wisher, S., & Klaber Moffatt, J. (2001). Barriers to Implementing the Evidence Base in Four NHS Therapies. *Physiotherapy*. 87, (8) 433-441.

Melton (2002). Occupational Therapy Service Strategy for Service Development and Research Programme. Gloucestershire Partnership NHS Trust.

NHS Centre for Review and Dissemination (1999) Effective health care, getting evidence into practice, The Royal Society of Medicine Press, University of York.

Roberts A. E. (2002). Advancing practice through continuing education: The case for reflection. *British Journal of Occupational Therapy*, 65 (5) 237-41.

Sackett D. L., Rosenberg W. M. C., Muir Gray J. A., Haynes R. B., & Richardson W. S. (1996). Evidence-based medicine: What it is and what it isn't. *British Medical Journal*, 312: 71-72.

Schon, D. A. (1991). The Reflective Practitioner: How Professionals Think in Action. England, Ashgate Publishing Ltd.

Scottish Executive (2002). *Building on Success: Future directions for the allied health professions in Scotland.*

Sleep, J., Page, S., & Tamblin, L. (2002). Achieving clinical excellence through evidence-based practice: Report of an educational initiative. *Journal of Nursing Management*, 10, 139-143.

Index

Numbers followed by "f" indicate figures; "t" following a page number indicates tabular material.

AAMR/Arc, Behavioral Supports policy statement of, 170
AARP Magazine, 38
Abreu, B.C., 96
Academic-clinical partnership(s), implications for practitioners as part of, 142-143
Academic-clinician partnership(s), future plans for, 104
Academic-Clinician Partnership model, 97-100
  collaborative process for benefits and challenges of, 103
    establishment of, 100-101
  development of, 97-99
  evaluation of, 103-104
  implementation of, 100-104
  structure of, 99-100
Academic-clinician partnerships, 95-106
Academic-practice partnership, in promotion of scholarship of "Best Practices," 71-93. *See also* Practice-Scholar Program
Access Living (AL), 58-63
  activities for entering, 59
  comparing CIL history and theory with OT in, 60-61
  described, 58-59
  describing of community partners in, 58-59
  promoting cultural competence in, 59-60

Accredited Educational Program for the Occupational Therapist (ACOTE), 98
ACOTE. *See* Accredited Educational Program for the Occupational Therapist (ACOTE)
Aging States Project, 42
AL. *See* Access Living (AL)
Allegheny County Department of Health and Human Services, 198
Allegheny County Jail, 82,194
  Department of OT at Duquesne University and, education and practice collaborations between, pilot study, 193-210
    described, 197-200
    instruments in, 201-203-208,207t-208t
    methods in, 200-203,202t
    procedures in, 203
    results of, 204-208,205t-208t
    subjects in, 201,202t
  inmates of, demographics of, 201,202t
Allegheny County Jail Community Re-entry Project, 198
Allegheny County Jail Community Re-Integration Project, 79
American Occupational Therapy Association Commission on Education, 124
AMPS. *See* Assessment of Motor and Process Skills (AMPS)
Apte, A., 173

Archstone Award, 39
Assessment of Communication and
    Interaction Skills, 24
Assessment of Motor and Process
    Skills (AMPS), 24,168

Barnett, R., 8
Before and After School Program, 64
Behavioral Supports policy statement,
    of AAMR/Arc, 170
Benson, J., 71
"Best Practices," scholarship of,
    promotion of,
    academic-practice
    partnership in, 71-93. See
    also Practice-Scholar
    Program
Bethlehem Haven, 79,81,82
BHI, Inc.. See Boston Health
    Interventions (BHI), Inc.
Birch, D.E., 147
Black Pride, 60
Bloomer, J.S., 96,98
Boston Health Interventions (BHI),
    Inc., 39
Boston University, National Institute
    of Aging-Funded Roybal
    Center for the Enhancement
    of Late-Life Function at, 33
Boston University Roybal Center
    (BURC), 33
Boyce, W., 147
Boyer, E.L., 75,76,124,131
Braveman, B., 11,147,173
BURC. See Boston University Roybal
    Center (BURC)
BURCELLF team, 36-42, 37t,40t

Campus Compact, 75,76
Canadian Occupational Performance
    Measure (COPM), 168
Carnegie Foundation, 75

Casas-Byots, C., 145
Center for Independent Living (CIL),
    166
    partnering and promoting praxis
    with, 58-63
Centre for Outcomes Research and
    Education, at UIC, 20
Certified OT assistants (COTAs), 91
CFS. See Chronic fatigue syndrome
    (CFS)
Chronic fatigue syndrome (CFS),
    116-117
CIL. See Center for Independent
    Living (CIL)
CIMT. See Constraint-induced
    movement therapy (CIMT)
Client(s), perceptions of OPTI-II,
    173-192. See also
    Occupational Performance
    History Interview–Second
    version (OPHI-II), therapists'
    and clients' perceptions of
CMH. See Community Mental Health
    (CMH)
Cockburn, L., 147
Cohn, E.S., 166
Collaborative partnership,
    development of, 151
Collaborative scholarly project,
    123-133. See also
    Constraint-induced
    movement therapy (CIMT)
Collaborative scholarship, background
    for, 124-125
College campus living, interagency
    collaboration in support of
    adults with developmental
    disabilities in, 165-171. See
    also Life Skills Experience
Community(ies), new resource to
    benefit, 77-78
Community Health Services, 40
Community Mental Health (CMH),
    166

Community Occupational Therapy, 146

Community Program Development model, 135-143. *See also* New Doors Model

Community Residential Corporation (CRC), 166

Community Television Network, 41

"Community University Conversation," 82

Competence, cultural, promotion of, in Access Living, 59-60

Conceptual framework, strategies for, 35-36
    application to MOB program, 36-42,37t,40t
    dissemination strategies, 36-42,37t,40t
    strategies targeted to OT clinicians
        embedding-related, 39
        experience-related, 38
        expertise-related, 38-39
        exposure-related, 36-38,37t

Concerns Report Methodology (CRM), 148
    action planning and action taken in, 156-157
    advocacy and learning training in, 156
    brainstorming ideas and identifying solutions in, 154-155
    concerns survey in, 152-153
    data analysis in, 153-154
    develop planning committees in, 156
    identification of community health service needs in, 152-154
    implications for community OT scholarship and practice, 157-158
    interviewers' training and data collection in, 153
    monitoring and feedback in, 157
    participants' characteristics in, 154
    phases of, 152-157,155t

plan and take action in, 156-157
    reflection on values and service needs in, 152
    service needs in, 154
    survey distribution in, 153

Constraint-induced movement therapy (CIMT), 123-133
    described, 128-130
    introduction to, 124

Consumer(s), New Doors Model implications for, 143

Continuum of care
    conceptualization of, 136-137
    defined, 136

Cooperative knowledge generation, interdisciplinary models of, 10-11

COPM. *See* Canadian Occupational Performance Measure (COPM)

COTAs. *See* Certified OT assistants (COTAs)

County jail practitioners, university faculty and, education and practice collaborations between, pilot study, 193-210
    discussion of, 208-209
    introduction to, 195-200
    problem/need in, 195-196

County jail practitioners, university faculty and, education and practice collaborations between, pilot study. *See also* Allegheny County Jail, Department of OT at Duquesne University and, education and practice collaborations between, pilot study

CRC. *See* Community Residential Corporation (CRC)

Creek, J., 18

Crist, P., 5,43-44,71,193

CRM. *See* Concerns Report Methodology (CRM)

Cultural competence, promotion of, in
     Access Living, 59-60
Cusick, A., 18

Dalhousie University, 96-97
Davidson, D.A., 167
Department of Health and Human
     Services (DHHS), 80
Department of Human Services, 63
Department of OT
   at Duquesne University, 194
   at UIC, 109
Department of OT faculty, at
     Duquesne University, 72,117
Developmental disabilities, college
     campus living and,
     interagency collaboration in
     support of, 165-171. *See also*
     Life Skills Experience (LSE)
DHHS. *See* Department of Health and
     Human Services (DHHS)
Dickerson, A., 2
Disability(ies)
   defined, 61-62
   developmental, college campus
     living and, interagency
     collaboration in support of,
     165-171. *See also* Life Skills
     Experience
Domestic violence community agency,
     building relationship with,
     63-66
Duncan, E.A.S., 17
Duquesne University,
     2,71,73,74,75,78,85,89
   Department of OT at. *See*
        Department of OT at
        Duquesne University
   Department of OT faculty at, 72
   new resource to benefit, 77-78
   Practice-Scholar Program at, 1

Eastern Michigan University (EMU),
     166,169,170

EBPP. *See* Evidence-based training
     programs (EBPP)
Education, New Doors Model
     implications for, 143
EE. *See* Empowerment evaluation
     (EE)
Eggers, M., 193
Embedding strategies, in conceptual
     framework, 35-36
Empowerment, defined, 62-63
Empowerment evaluation (EE), 11-12
EMU. *See* Eastern Michigan
     University (EMU)
"Enabling Self-Determination (ESD)
     for people living with AIDS,"
     177
Eraut, M., 8
Evashwick, C., 137
Evidence-based interventions, model
     for dissemination and
     utilization of, 31-46
   conceptual framework for, 35-36
   introduction to, 32
   recommendations for, 42-43
   strategies for, 35-36
Evidence-based practice
   achieving of, 211-227. *See also*
        GPT/UKCORE partnership;
        United Kingdom Centre for
        Outcomes research and
        Education (UK CORE), GPT
        and, partnership between
   background of, 212-213
   defined, 212
   delivery of
      building structures in support of,
        by UKCORE with TSH,
        22-26,25f
      evidence of, 26,27f
   evaluation of, 224-226,225f
   identifying trainers in, 221
   implementation of, 218-220
   rationale for, 212-213
   reflections in, 224-226,225f
   role definition in, 220-221

role development in, trainer
meetings in support of,
221-223,222f,223f
supporting accountability as trainer
in, 224
time to deliver trainer role in, 223
Evidence-based practice training
programme
content of, 215-217,216t
implementation of, 218-220
problem identification in,
214-218,215t,216t
process of building, 214
structure of, 217-218
Evidence-based training programs
(EBPP), development of, 213
Experience strategies, in conceptual
framework, 35
Expertise strategies, in conceptual
framework, 35
Exposure strategies, in conceptual
framework, 35

Fairman, A., 193
Family Independence Agency (FIA),
166
Family Rescue, 63,64
Farkas, M., 31
Fawcett, S.B., 149
FIA. *See* Family Independence Agency
(FIA)
Finlayson, M., 9,148
Fisher, G., 107
Fitzgerald, L., 167
Forsyth, K., 13,17,203,211
Freire, P., 49,149

Gay Pride, 60
Gloucestershire Partnership NHS Trust
(GPT)
described, 213

UK CORE and, partnership
between, 211-227. *See also*
GPT/UKCORE partnership
Good Beginnings Program, 78-79,81
Goodwill Industries of Pittsburgh,
79,81-82,194,197
GPT. *See* Gloucestershire Partnership
NHS Trust (GPT)
GPT/UKCORE partnership, 211-227
background of, 212-213
evaluation of, 224-226,225f
identifying trainers in, 221
problem identification in,
214-218,215t,216t
process of building, 214
rationale for, 212-213
reflections in, 224-226,225f
role definition in, 220-221
role development in, trainer
meetings in support of,
221-223,222f,223f
supporting accountability as trainer
in, 224
time to deliver trainer role in, 223
Gray, C.M., 165
Great Cities mission, 110,111
Greenfield, L., 195

Hadley, J., 159
Hall, M., 167
Hammel, J., 9,11,47,109,147
Hansen, A.M.W., 1,71,193
Hargraves, J.L., 159
Head Start, 63
Head-Ball, D., 47
Healthviews, 41
Healthy People 2010 goals, 137
Heine, D.M., 165
Helfrich, C., 9,47
Hispanic immigrants, health services
needs of, identification of,
PAR approach in, 145-163

Home Management Skills Program
        Evaluation project, 101-103
Howland, J., 31

ICP. *See* Integrated care pathway (ICP)
"Illinois Plan," 109
ILS. *See* Independent living skills
        (ILS)
Immigrant(s), Hispanic, health services
        needs of, PAR approach to,
        145-163
Incarceration, OT in, research on,
        196-197
Independence, defined, 61-62
Independent living skills (ILS),
        defined, 166
Institutional Review Board (IRB),
        99,101,126,177
Integrated care pathway (ICP), 23-24
Interest Checklist, 114
IRB. *See* Institutional Review Board
        (IRB)

Johnson, C., 135
Jones, E.J., 197
Jose-Kampfner, C., 204
Journal of Physical Activity and Aging,
        42

Kean University, 97
Kean University Institutional Research
        Board, 101
Kean University Occupational Therapy
        faculty, 97-98
Kearns, J.F., 167
Kielhofner, G.,
        5,7,9,13,43-44,107,114,173,
        176,203
Kleinert, H.L., 167
Knowledge creating systems, 12-13

Langile, L., 147
Langley, J., 147
Lewin, K., 49
Life Skills Experience, 165-171
    background of, 166-167
    literature review of, 167-168
    method of, 168-169
    recommendations for, 170
London South Bank University, 20
Ludwig-Beymer, P., 152-153
Lysack, C., 143,147

MacKinnon, C., 8
Mahaffey, L., 176
Maine Medical Center, 40-41
MaineHealth, 39,40
MaineHealth Learning Resource
        Center, 41
Mallinson, T., 176
Mann, L.S., 211
Martinez, L.I., 145
Master of occupational therapy
        (MOTO), 125
Mathews, R.M., 149
Matter of balance (MOB) program, 41
        application of conceptual
                framework to, 36-42,37t,40t
        evaluation of, 32-34
        origins of, 32-34
McCluskey, A., 18
McColl, M.A., 167,197
McMahon, E.W., 31
Melton, J., 211
*Mental Health Special Interest
        Quarterly,* 86
Mercy College, 97
Metcalf, C., 18
Michigan Campus Venture Grant, 166
Miller, K.S., 131
Minority Group Model, 60
MOB Facilitator Training Manual,
        38-39
MOB program. *See* Matter of balance
        (MOB) program

Model of Human Occupation
(MOHO),
19,23,113,114,115,118,201,
203-208,207t-208t
Model of Human Occupation (MOHO)
Clearinghouse, 115
MOHO. *See* Model of Human
Occupation (MOHO)
MOTO. *See* Master of occupational
therapy (MOTO)
Movement therapy, constraint-induced,
123-133. *See also*
Constraint-induced
movement therapy (CIMT)
Munoz, J.P., 71,193

National Health Service (NHS), 19,213
National Institute of Aging-Funded
Roybal Center for the
Enhancement of Late-Life
Function, at Boston
University, 33
National Institutes of Child Health and
Human Development, 117
National Public Radio's broadcast, 38
Native American Maliseet tribe, 42
Neidstadt, M.E., 166
New Doors Model, 135-143
described, 136,137-140,140t
implications for education, 143
implications for OT practice,
142-143
implications for potential
consumers, 143
implications for practitioners as part
of academic-clinical
partnership, 142-143
literature review of, 136-137
outcomes of, 141-142
phase one of, 138-139,140t
phase three of, 139-140,140t
phase two of, 139,140t
New Freedom Initiative, 167
New York Times, 38

NHS organization. *See* National Health
Service (NHS) organization
1998 American Public Health
Association Archstone
Foundation Award for
Excellence in Program
Innovation, 37

OCAIRS. *See* Occupational
Circumstances Interview and
Rating Scale (OCAIRS)
Occupational Circumstances Interview
and Rating Scale (OCAIRS),
24
Occupational Performance History
Interview, 114
Occupational Performance History
Interview–Second version
(OPHI-II)
administration of, 175,175f
introduction to, 174
narrative slope of
client participant perspectives
on, 186-188,186f
perceptions of, 180-183
previous research on, 175-176
therapists' and clients' perceptions
of, 173-192
study of
aims of, 176
context of, 177
data collection in, 178
discussion of, 189-190
findings of, 178-179
impact of interview process on,
185-186
influence of client characteristics
on, 179-180
methods in, 177-178
participants in, 177-178
perceptions in, 179
perceptions of, 184-186
sampling, 177-178

Occupational Self Assessment (OSA), 24,114,168,194,201,203-208, 207t-208t
Occupational therapy (OT), in incarceration, research on, 196-197
Occupational Therapy (OT) Department, 76
Occupational therapy (OT) practice, New Doors Model implications for, 142-143
Occupational therapy (OT) scholarship and practice, university-community partnerships for
building and maintaining of, 51-57,52f
building cultural competence in, 55-56
building entry and competence in, 50-51
developing reciprocal learning opportunities in, 52-53
developing relationship based on trust and mutual respect in, 51-52,52f
establishing open lines of communication in, 53
exemplars of, 58-66
impact of, 57-58
maximizing resources in, 54-55
model of, 47-70
outcomes of, 57-58
respecting diversity in, 55-56
sharing accountability in, 56-57
using multi-method approach to scholarship and practice in, 55
Occupational therapy (OT) service case study, in United Kingdom, 17-29
background of, 18-20
introduction to, 18-19
rationale for, 18-20

Occupational therapy (OT) SoP, CRM implications for, 157-158
Office of Research on Women's Health, 117
Olmstead Act, 167
OPTI-II. See Occupational Performance History Interview–Second version (OPHI-II)
OSA. See Occupational Self Assessment (OSA)
OT. See Occupational therapy (OT)
OT Practice, 86
OTHC, 2
Ottenbacher, K., 96

PAR. See Participatory Action Research (PAR)
Participatory Action Research (PAR), 49
Participatory action research (PAR) background of, 149,151
CRM as, 148-149
in identification of health service needs of Hispanic immigrants, 145-163
Participatory research (PR), 145-163
Partnership, collaborative, development of, 151
Partnership for Healthy Aging (PFHA), 39,40-42,40t
Paul-Ward, A., 173
Peloquin, S.M., 96
Peterson, E.W., 9,31
Petty, R., 149
PFHA. See Partnership for Healthy Aging (PFHA)
Pollock, N., 130
PR. See Participatory research (PR)
Practice, scholarship and, coupling of, barriers to, 8-9
Practice scholar(s), developing of, 84-86

Practice-scholar outcomes, 86,87t-88t
Practice-Scholar Program, 71-93
    background of, 75-77
    creating new internal structure to
        support, 82-83
    described, 78-80
    at Duquesne University, 1
    fieldwork development in, 89
    funding of, 83-84,83t
    future goals of, 91
    identification of suitable partners,
        80-82
    instructional innovation in, 88
    new developments in, 91
    outcomes of, 86,87t-88t
    programmatic transitions and
        modifications in, 90-91
    student engagement in,
        87t-88t,89-90
Practitioner-academic partnership,
        continuing education through
        process of, 211-227. *See also*
        GPT/UKCORE partnership;
        United Kingdom Centre for
        Outcomes Research and
        Education (UK CORE), GPT
        and, partnership between
Prilleltensky, I., 149
Project Employ program, 79
Provident, I., 71

Ramsay, D., 158
Reflection, in GPT/UKCORE
        partnership, 224-226,225f
Reflective Practitioner, 75
REIS. *See* Residential Environment
        Impact Survey (REIS)
Research, participatory, 145-163
Residential Environment Impact
        Survey (REIS), 113,115
Resources for Human Development
        (RHD), 141
RHD. *See* Resources for Human
        Development (RHD)

Robertson, S.C., 158
Rochon, S., 130
Rose, J.F., 165
Roybal Center, 42
Roybal website, 36

SAOF. *See* Self-Assessment of
        Occupational Functioning
        (SAOF)
Scharmer, 12,13
Scholarly project process,
        125-128,127t
Scholarship, practice and, coupling of,
        barriers to, 8-9
Scholarship of practice (SoP)
    building of, process of,
        20-26,21f,25f
    cycle of, completing of, 31-46. *See
        also* Evidence-based
        interventions, model for
        dissemination and utilization
        of
    described, 32,109-112,111f
    introduction to, 32
    OT, CRM implications for, 157-158
    outcomes of, 26-28,27f
    partnerships for, developing and
        maintaining of, 50
    at UIC, 1
    in United Kingdom, 17-29. *See also*
        Occupational therapy (OT)
        service case study, in United
        Kingdom
Scholarship of Practice (SoP) model,
        synthesizing research,
        education, and practice
        according to, faculty
        examples of, 107-122
    clinical track faculty member,
        112-116
    research-track faculty member,
        116-120
Scholarship practice gap, 8-13
Scholarship Reconsidered, 75

Schriner, K.F., 149
Sciulli, J., 193
Sclön, D., 75
Selener, D., 156
Self-Assessment of Occupational
    Functioning (SAOF), 203
Senge, 12,13
Social Model of Disability, 60
SoP. *See* Scholarship of practice (SoP)
Southern Maine Agency on Aging, 40
Staff Development Self-Assessment,
    114
Stern, K.A., 95
Stern, P., 104
Stube, J., 123
Suarez-Balcazar, Y., 47,50,145
Summerfield-Mann, L., 13,17

Taylor, R.R.. 11,107,147
The State Hospital (TSH), 18
    UKCORE and, partnership
        between, 20-26,21f,25f. *See
        also* United Kingdom Centre
        for Outcomes Research and
        Education (UKCORE), TSH
        with, partnership between
    Therapist(s), perceptions of
        OPTI-II, 173-192. *See also*
        Occupational Performance
        History Interview–Second
        version (OPHI-II), therapists'
        and clients' perceptions of
Thomas, J., 47
Townsend, E., 147
Transitional Housing Program, 64
Trentham, B., 147
TSH. *See* The State Hospital (TSH)
TSH/UKCORE partnership. *See*
    United Kingdom Centre for
    Outcomes Research and
    Education (UKCORE), TSH
    with
2002 World Federation of
    Occupational Therapy, 1

UIC. *See* University of
    Illinois–Chicago (UIC)
UKCORE. *See* United Kingdom
    Centre for Outcomes
    Research and Education
    (UKCORE)
UND. *See* University of North Dakota
    (UND)
United Kingdom
    OT service case study in, 17-29. *See
        also* Occupational therapy
        (OT) service case study, in
        United Kingdom
    SoP in, 17-29. *See also*
        Occupational therapy (OT)
        service case study, in United
        Kingdom
United Kingdom Centre for Outcomes
    Research and Education (UK
    CORE)
    described, 213
    GPT and, partnership between,
        211-227. *See also*
        GPT/UKCORE partnership
United Kingdom Centre for Outcomes
    Research and Education
    (UKCORE), 18,20
    described, 19-20
    TSH with
        building structures to support
            delivering of evidence-based
            practice by, 22-26,25f
        described, 20-21
        evidence-based assessment
            protocols of, 24-25
        evidence-based development
            groups for staff in, 26
        ICP in, 23-24
        initial negotiations, 21-22
        leadership in, 25-26
        managerial structures of,
            23-26,25f
        parameters of, 23
        partnership between,
            20-26,21f.25f

practice changes in, evidence of,
26,27f
practitioners generating
evidence for practice in,
27-28
R&D strategic document of, 23
strategic planning by, 22-23
supervision structures of, 25
University of Illinois Hospital, 110
University of Illinois–Chicago (UIC),
9,28,50,63,76,97,108-109,
116
approach to education at, 111
approach to scholarship at, 110-111
approach to service at, 111-112
. Centre for Outcomes Research and
Education at, 20
Department of Occupational
Therapy at, 109
integrating scholarship, education,
and service at, 112
IRB of, 177
SoP at, 1
University of Kansas, 148
University of North Dakota (UND),
124,125,126,128
University of Southern Maine, 40
University-community partnerships,
for OT scholarship and
practice, 47-70. *See also*
Occupational therapy (OT)
scholarship and practice,
university-community
partnerships for

Velde, B.P., 55,158
Violence, domestic, community
agency for, building
relationship with, 63-66

WACA. *See* Washtenaw Association
for Community Advocacy
(WACA)
Waddock, S., 73,74
Wade, B.D., 109
Walsh, M., 73,74
Washtenaw Association for
Community Advocacy
(WACA), 166
Washtenaw Intermediate School
District (WISD), 166,168,169
Whiteford, 197
WIA funding program, 80
Widman Foundation, 166
Wilcock, A., 196
Wilson, T., 47
WISD. *See* Washtenaw Intermediate
School District (WISD)
Wister Street Project, 141
Wittman, P.P., 55,158
Wolf Motor Function Test, 129
Work Incentive Act (WIA) funding
program, 80
Work Role Interview, 24-25

Y-Care Day Care, 79
YMCA of Pittsburgh, 79,81

Printed and bound by CPI Group (UK) Ltd, Croydon, CR0 4YY

17/10/2024

01775687-0005